THE BENEFITS OF TOBACCO

The Surprising Therapeutic Effects of Moderate Smoking and Second Hand Smoke

A Smoker's Paradox

William Campbell Douglass II, MD
Tracy T. Douglass, Editor and Researcher

Rhino Publishing, S.A.

THE HEALTH BENEFITS OF TOBACCO

Copyright ©
by

William Campbell Douglass II, MD

Cover Illustration by
Alex Manyoma
alex@3dcity.com

Book Layout by
Lourdes Jaramillo
lourja@cwpanama.net

Back Cover, Layout and Design by
David Mitty
freelancelife@aol.com

Please, visit www.drtobacco.com to order this book
and for other publications from
Dr. William Campbell Douglass and Rhino Publishing.

Dr. Douglass' "Real Health" alternative medical newsletter is
available at www.realhealthnews.com

RHINO PUBLISHING, S.A.
World Trade Center
Panama, Republic of Panama

Voicemail/Fax
International: + 416-352-5126
North America: 888-317-6767

To all the

Beleaguered

Persecuted

and

Humiliated

smokers of the world, don't worry,
you are not killing people with
side-stream smoke... <u>people</u> are killing:

Liberty

Common Sense

Fairness

and

Constitutional Rights

all in the name of

Science.

William Campbell Douglass II, MD

Acknowledgements

There were numerous sources sited and reprinted in this book. We would like to thank everyone who agreed to contribute and also thank them for their dedication to uncovering the truth surrounding this important issue.

A special acknowledgement goes to the following people:

Marc J. Schneiderman MD
Dr. John A. Rosecrans PhD
Joseph Perkins
Dr. Gio Batta Gori
Tom (author "Developing Ideas" Montalk)
Dr. Hugh Tunstall Pedoe
Dr. John Gofman

We also give a very special thanks to FORCES International and their volunteer staff (listed below) of talented and informed contributors and writers. I have quoted and extracted numerous writings from Forces International and without their findings and compiled information this book would not have been possible. Please visit their web site at www.forces.org for an in-depth look at the conspiracy, and fraud surrounding the anti-smoking campaign:

Carol Thompson
Wanda Hamilton
Joy Faulkner
Gian Turci

Table of Contents

"The evidence is clear.
A moderate amount of smoking
is an avenue to good health
and to the prevention of a variety of diseases."

Dr. Tobacco

Introduction

The Oxford English Dictionary defines <u>paradox</u>:

"A statement or tenet contrary to received opinion or belief...as being discordant with what is held to be established truth, and hence absurd or fantastic."

So every time you light up, you can remember it for your smoking pleasure *"the smokers paradox"*. What could be more absurd or fantastic than the <u>smoker's</u> paradox -- *Smoking in moderation for a healthy life while he is being told that he is killing himself!*

The following quote is a good summary of the illogical and dishonest media the smoker faces: "Since the benefits of smoking are too numerous and consistent to be attributable to error or random chance, it follows that the "<u>established truth</u>", asserting that smoking is the cause of (almost) all disease cannot be true - a reality that dramatically clashes with the gigantic corruption of public health, its pharmaceutical and insurance mentors, institutions and media." (Quoted from *Forces*, the British defenders of the right to smoke)

Ref: http://www.forces.org/evidence/evid/therap.htm

I must confess that I did not expect to find the broad spectrum of therapeutic and preventive applications of tobacco smoke for human medicine. In the early years of my practice, I was such a fanatic on the subject of cigarette smoking that I would refuse to continue to treat a patient who would not quit smoking.

My only positive attitudes toward smoking were a fondness for cigars, their tendency to discourage the presence of neurotic, overly sensitive and garrulous female types, and the observation that my cigar-smoking patients and friends lived long, healthy lives. (This is not meant to be an indictment of all women. Some of my best friends are women and some of them, even on occasion, smoke a cigar.)

The benefits of smoking tobacco have been known since ancient times, from sharpening mental acuity to maintaining optimal weight. The relatively small risks of smoking have always been outweighed by the substantial improvement to mental and physical health. The reasons for this are unclear. It probably has to do with the beneficial effects of carbon monoxide (in small doses) and other effects still unknown.

Tobacco has been used for a variety of medicinal purposes. Topically, it has been employed to treat wounds. Internally, it has been used to treat gastric disorders, and it was often used as an anti-depressant. Today, cigar smokers use it to embrace feelings of relaxation, clarity, stimulation, and creativity.

The "full court press" against smokers began in the 70s. It started in what you might say was a positive way, at least as far as insurance was concerned. Restaurants were also even handed in that they offered non-smoking areas for patrons who disliked smoke. No one complained about that, because it was obviously fair. But now, the situation is reversed. The next stage was to have <u>smoking</u> areas, rather than <u>non-smoking</u> areas and now many restaurants don't allow smoking at all. There are also non-smoking hotels and non-smoking ships! Florida purists, moralists, and environmental wackos want to make Florida the first non-smoking <u>state</u>!

The anti-tobacco fanatics are in a tough spot. Reliable scientific research has turned up the horrible news that tobacco smoke is good for your health. Alzheimer's, Parkinson's, Tourette's Syndrome, and Senile Brain Disease are among some diseases that can be alleviated or even cured by tobacco. There is even evidence that tobacco helps to prevent colon and prostate cancer. The drug industry is scrambling to capitalize on this good news by promoting the nicotine patch. So the same industry that has been saying that nicotine is bad for you in any shape has changed its mind. It's OK to put nicotine into your system so long as you do it <u>our</u> way – through the skin and not the lungs. The positive revelations regarding tobacco will not go away and are very good reasons to keep lighting those cigars and cigarettes – <u>in moderation</u>.

Ref: http://193.78.190.200/10/nicoplus.htm   Nicotine Drugs Hold Promise for Treating Neurological Disease Alzheimer's patients may benefit, scientists say.

Could there really be ANY health benefits to tobacco?

You've heard the other side of the story until you can't imagine there being <u>any</u> health benefits from nicotine and the herb from which it comes -- tobacco. You are in for a surprise, which I hope, will awaken you to the fact that the news media can "lie" by simply not reporting the research presenting the good side on a food or herb that is not politically correct. On the other hand, they will not report (or they will put it in size six type) the bad side of something that is part of the liberal/medical establishment agenda, such as fluoride, NSAIDS (Non Steroidal Anti-Inflammatory Drugs) and soy "milk."

<u>Let me state here that I am not endorsing the smoking of cigarettes</u>. When you inhale smoke from cigarettes – and 99 percent of habitual cigarette smokers DO inhale – you are not only pulling hundreds of <u>hot</u> chemicals into the delicate alveoli of your lungs but you are inhaling the smoke of <u>burning paper</u>. People seldom think about the paper, which may be the most detrimental element in cigarette smoking. No one actually knows how harmful the paper is and it would be difficult to research it, but even cigarettes, if smoked in moderation – less than ten a day – have been <u>proven harmless</u>.

Good quality cigars from Central America contain only tobacco, unlike the trash produced in Tampa and other American cities. The only exception to this that I know of is Reno Nevada, there may be other places. The wrapper, the outside cover that holds the cigar together, is high-quality tobacco leaf, not paper. There is no paper and no additives of any kind added to the construction of a good cigar. Highly trained experts make their quality cigars by hand and almost all of them smoke while working. Even though they're exposed all day to damp tobacco leaves, as they are rolled with bare hands (see center photo album), they live a normal, healthy life. Their rate of cancer and heart disease is no different from the general population, and **as you will learn from reading this book,** there is a remarkable <u>positive</u> side to tobacco exposure in moderate doses.

While it is true that you can get many benefits by smoking cigarettes (and there are many listed in this book) they <u>are</u> toxic! IF you smoke more than half a pack per day, at the very least you will get chronic purulent bronchitis, and probably emphysema, and maybe lung cancer. To be on the safe side I recommend a maximum of six to ten cigarettes a day, but if you have never smoked, you will find smoking and inhaling to be an unpleasant experience.

There are four practical alternatives to cigarette smoking: cigars, pipe smoking, the nicotine patch, and the water pipe. Although not as convenient, the water pipe is a nontoxic and benign method for getting your nicotine requirement. If you want to go the "clean" way, the water pipe is the choice for you.

SECTION I

THE DISEASES
AND THE EVIDENCE

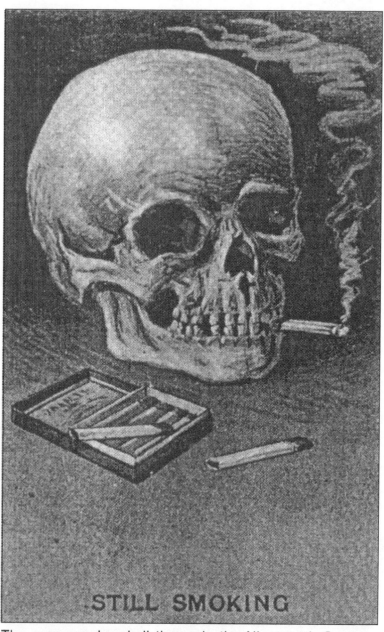

STILL SMOKING

The ever-popular skull theme in the Nineteenth Century. Apparently, smoking didn't destroy your teeth until the Twentieth Century.

The Proof is in the Puffing

Enough political polemics, let's look at the scientific evidence that supports the use of tobacco for health reasons. If you have heard enough and want only the bare facts, go to the Appendix and read *"Environmental Tobacco Smoke and Coronary Heart Syndromes: Absence of an Association."* This report is from *Regulatory Toxicology and Pharmacology* 21, 281-295 (1995). It's REAL SCIENCE and makes the case for the puffers. After reading this, you will not have to read the rest of this book (but no refunds). Following is a section on diseases and their association with tobacco.

Ref: Regulatory Toxicology and Pharmacology 21, 281-295 (1995).

CHAPTER 1
Heart

A Contrary Study - without Merit

The following study is a contrary view to the hypotheses of this book. This issue – smoking and coronary heart disease -- is not resolved by any means. But there is something that continues to nag me about these studies: They talk about smoking without really quantifying <u>the dosage</u> of smoke the patients are receiving. In fact, it probably would be impossible to do so.

My point is important: Could anyone, except the most fanatical tobacco-phobics, object to a person smoking six cigarettes or three cigars a day for health reasons, especially since the research clearly shows that a little smoke is a good thing?

Hasdai and colleagues (Effect of smoking status on the long-term outcome after successful percutaneous coronary re-vascularization), New England Journal of Medicine, 1997; 336(11) came to the following conclusion concerning "smoking" (whatever that may imply since they don't know how many cigarettes the individual actually smoked): There is a significant "clinical" improvement in smokers who continue to smoke after angioplasty but, they claim, angiograms show no difference between smoker and non-smoker after the surgery: "Although smokers experienced a 31% reduction in clinical restenosis, ...paradoxically there were no differences in angiographic restenosis or other angiographic parameters at follow-up." Since angiograms are <u>notoriously inaccurate</u>, not related to the clinical condition of the patient, and not reproducible, these findings are without significance. The only thing their study proved is that "...smokers experience a 31% reduction in clinical restenosis."

It should be added that the investigators do not attempt to deny that there was "a reduction in clinical restenosis" associated with smoking. They merely say that the reduction "is not due to a reduction in <u>angiographic</u> restenosis." (i.e., not demonstrable by angiography.) To me, this appears to be a deliberate obfuscation of the <u>good</u> news – <u>smokers have a 31 percent reduction in the necessity to have the operation repeated</u>.

The authors wonder out loud if their results might be an example of "angiographic-clinical dissociation," that is, a high class example of the "smokers' paradox." They conclude that, because of the excellence of their study, there is no paradox. Well, I beg to differ. There is dissociation between what was found by observation of the patient and other tests as opposed to the results of angiographic studies. That is because angiography is not a "gold standard" as is claimed, but a pretended one. They should not be used to distort the obvious: <u>Moderate smoking is good for patients with cardiovascular disease</u>.

Furthermore, if the investigators do not know the dosage of smoke (nicotine) the subjects have had, how can they come to any conclusion at all? Frequent blood nicotine levels or cotinine levels would be essential for a truly scientific study.

See appendix: A Contrary Study without Merit.

Cardiovascular Disease and Infection

"You can't find what you don't look for" is a popular adage in medical research. Researchers had become so convinced that smoking was a major cause of heart disease they ignored evidence that bacterial infection seems to play a major role. If the deceased was a heavy smoker, then why look further? But as more researchers look for evidence of chronic infection in the heart and arteries, the more they see. It has gotten to the point that the pathologist better do tissue studies or he will be criticized. Tobacco has taken most of the heat, along with (innocent) cholesterol and (innocent) animal fat. Another culprit that has been ignored is fluoride, which is probably even more of a risk than homocysteine (folic acid, B12, and B6 deficiency).

Let's pursue this a little further so that you can see that the scientific evidence is compelling --they don't find <u>nicotine</u> in these diseased arteries, they find <u>BUGS</u>.

Epidemiologic studies have demonstrated an association between serologic evidence of *Chlamydia pneumoniae* infection and atherosclerotic disease of the coronary and other arteries. In addition, *C. pneumoniae* <u>has been identified in atherosclerotic plaques</u> by electron microscopy. Recently, the organism has also been recovered <u>in culture</u> from atheromatous plaque. This indicates the presence of <u>viable replicating bacteria</u> in the vessels. Animal studies support the hypothesis that *C. pneumoniae* infection of the upper respiratory tract is followed by recovery of the organism from atheromatous lesions in the aorta and that <u>the infection accelerates the process of atherosclerosis</u>.

So the question you are about to ask me is: "Should I take a course of antibiotics occasionally as a preventive?" In some cases, perhaps yes. My answer may surprise you but I am only referring to patients at <u>extreme risk</u> – those with unstable angina, or recent heart attack, or both. Some investigators claim that antibiotic therapy <u>reverses the increased risk of atherosclerosis</u> in infected animals. If this is confirmed by further studies, it can have momentous implications on the treatment or prevention of cardiovascular disease. (Do I hear a great drooling noise coming from the boardrooms of the pharmaceutical industry?)

Two small trials in patients with unstable angina or recent myocardial infarction suggest that antibiotics will reduce subsequent cardiac events. Larger trials have been initiated to determine more definitively whether antibiotics affect the risk of atherosclerosis.

My point in reporting this to you is that <u>smoking is a red herring</u> in the quest for the cause and prevention of cardiovascular disease.

Action to take: Smoke three cigars a day and forget the antibiotics. (<u>Don't inhale</u>, your mucous membranes will absorb adequate nicotine for good health.)

See appendix: CVD and Infection.

Ref: Harrison's Textbook of Medicine, Chapter 242.

Fright Therapy

Researchers in the Seychelles and Switzerland reported at the annual meeting of the American College of Cardiology on the effect of smoking on the coronary arteries, blockage of which causes heart attacks, (or so they say). Photos of the effect of tobacco on the arteries, shocked many smokers into giving it up, they said.

Maybe we could shock more smokers into quitting by putting an angiographer in every shopping center. Trouble is, none of the shopping malls allow smoking any more. Easy solution: a sign that states: "<u>NO SMOKING </u>unless taking an angiogram."

"… It is very interesting to see that notwithstanding the sharp decrease in smoking, the rate of hospitalization for Coronary Heart Disease has actually increased. It is also interesting to see how the explanations for this "mystery" go in every possible direction, but the most instinctive and logical one is:

smoking does not cause CHD. But this would mean proving once again that the dogma dictating that tobacco is an absolute health evil is <u>false</u>, and this is, of course, not politically acceptable, for the government grant money and the support of the pharmaceutical industry might be seriously compromised."

Courtesy of Carol Thompson Smokers' Rights Action Group.
P.O. Box 259575 Madison, WI 53725-9575.

Is the Carbon Monoxide in Tobacco Smoke Beneficial?

The doctor of the future: "I TOLD you not to quit smoking!"

Much has been said about the carbon monoxide (CM) found in tobacco smoke. Carbon monoxide in sufficient amounts is deadly; there is no doubt about that. So is cobra venom and botulinum toxin, but in tiny amounts they have been found effective in certain conditions. CM has also been found to have significant medical benefits in tiny amounts. It's the new (to most people) science of hormesis.

It is interesting to note that public health doctors think it is OK to dose you on a continuous basis with fluoride in your water, even though the highly toxic fluoride is <u>cumulative in your tissues</u>, including your brain and CM is not. But "everyone knows" CM is a deadly gas (which it is) and so it cannot be used <u>in any amount</u> for medical purposes, which is contrary to all basic pharmacological principles and knowledge.

<u>This is the key</u> to the Luddite thinking of these simpletons, the black hole in the mind of the average Greenie fanatic, who can't understand that the "zero tolerance" attitude, if adhered to, would mean elimination of all salt in the diet, all spices, cows (prodigious producers of methane gas), all fluoride (good idea!) all industrialization, and the elimination of <u>every tree on earth</u>! Trees are one of the great pollution criminals. And say goodbye to your precious campfires and all windmills – a massive killer of birds. A little tobacco smoke, side stream or front stream, is a very good thing – LEARN TO LIVE WITH IT.

And now comes the mother of all medical shockers: <u>Tobacco smoke may alleviate heart attacks and stroke</u>.

Carbon monoxide is a by-product of tobacco smoke. A report indicates low levels of carbon monoxide may help victims of heart attacks and strokes.

Carbon monoxide inhibits blood clotting, thereby dissolving harmful clots in the arteries. The researchers focused on carbon monoxide's close resemblance to nitric oxide that keeps blood vessels from dilating and prevents the buildup of the detritus of clotting. The researchers commented: "Recently nitric oxide has been elevated from a common air pollutant... to an [internal] second messenger of utmost physiological importance. Therefore, many of us may not be entirely surprised to learn that carbon monoxide can... rescue the lung from [vascular] injury," reports the researchers.

The extrapolation from this is that cigar smoke can relieve ischemic heart disease through the minute amounts of carbon monoxide present.

Ref: The Carbon Monoxide Paradox: http://193.78.190.200/10b/cm.htm

A New Twist on "Roto-Ruter"
The Impact of Smoking on Preventing Reclosure of the Heart Arteries.

"Everybody" knows that smoking causes heart disease, i.e., a narrowing of the arteries of the heart. If this is true, then they'll have a hard time explaining the research reported below, no matter how hard they huff and puff.

There is a popular invasive procedure called angioplasty, which is basically a "Roto-Ruter" of the arteries of the heart. Restenosis, a subsequent replugging of the arteries, is all too common with this surgery.

This extensive study shows yet another benefit of smoking. Smokers have much better chances to survive, heal, and do well because they are less likely to experience restenosis than non-smokers. Even though it has been proven that moderate smoking, especially cigars, gives patients a better chance of surviving angioplasty, the people must not be told because they might get the idea that smoking may be good for them – a totally unacceptable paradox (AGAIN). You will not see this study reported in Reuters Health. This was a highly significant study and where is the press? Do you think you will ever see this headline: "People increase their chances of death from cardiovascular disease by not smoking."

Ref: Circulation, 2001,104, 773 – Therapeutic Effects of Smoking and Nicotine. "Impact of Smoking on Clinical and Angiographic Restenosis After Percutaneous Coronary Intervention".

http://193.78.190.200/34/circulation_2001_104_773.htm

Nicotine and Angiogenesis

<u>A Stanford scientist has been honored for his research indicating that nicotine holds potential for non-surgical heart by-pass procedures.</u>

Dr. Christopher Heeschen of Stanford University was honored by the American College of Cardiology for his research on the effect of nicotine on angiogenesis (new blood vessel growth). His work took third place in the year 2000 *Young Investigators Competition* in the category of Physiology, Pharmacology and Pathology. Dr. Heeschen presented compelling data from research done at Stanford revealing that the simple plant protein, nicotine, applied in small harmless doses, produced new blood vessel growth around blocked arteries to oxygen-starved tissue.

A company has been formed in Texas to exploit these findings, and their product is now being employed successfully around the world in the treatment of blocked heart arteries.

Ref: Nicotine Promotes Arteriogenesis.
     http://www.ncbi.nlm.nih.gov/entrez/query.fcgi?cmd=
     Retrieve&db=PubMed&list_uids=12575981&dopt=Abstract

Nicotine – the Fountain of Youth?

I don't think so! Nicotine, like so many other things, cures or kills, depending on <u>the dose</u>. That's basically the theme of this book. Nicotine can kill in large, continuous doses but, paradoxically, it holds great promise in heart cell regeneration – another example of the "Smokers' Paradox."

Endovasc Inc. of Montgomery, Texas, announced on Nov. 4, 2003, the results of their continuing work on therapy with nicotine in cardiovascular disease. They said that research conducted at the Texas Heart Institute, Heart Failure Research Lab, directed under Yong-Jian Geng, MD Ph. D., "indicated that nicotine has significant effects on both the proliferation and differentiation of mouse embryonic stem cells. We are narrowing the mechanistic action of nicotine that accelerates stem cell division while closing in on the signal transduction pathway underlying the process of myocardiogenesis" (the creation of new heart cells).

In his study, Dr. Geng used embryonic cardiac stem cells isolated from rodents cultured in special media to support their growth and development. In cultures treated with very low levels of nicotine, the rate of stem cell division increased significantly, compared to untreated cells. These new findings confirm and extend earlier studies conducted at Stanford University that support the growing theory that <u>nicotine can boost stem cell regenerative powers in patients with chronic or congestive heart failure</u>.

The Texas Heart Institute research team also performed adult stem cell transplantation for heart failure patients in collaboration with Brazilian cardiologists. (The results were not reported in the company press release from which this material was derived.)

So, while you are waiting for science to apply tobacco for the regeneration of your heart, damaged from the bad nutritional advice of the U.S. government and your cardiologist, light up three stogies daily but do not inhale – and that's not a bad Clinton joke, but this doctor's advice, based on 50 years of experience.

Ref: Press Release Endovasc, Inc. 11/04/03.

A Smoker with an Infected Heart --
Who, Gets Blamed for the Death?

It is now fairly well established that certain infectious organisms are related to heart disease, especially H. pylori and C. pneumoniae. Yet, when a diseased heart is the cause of death, and the patient was a smoker with evidence of a chronic infection, the history of smoking will be listed as the cause of death or at least a co-factor. This is impossible to prove and has skewed the statistics against smoking. Compounding the problem is the fact that infective organisms may be present in the tissues of the heart but were not discovered because the blood tested negative for antibodies to the organism. So the tissues of the heart were not examined for organisms and smoking got blamed as the cause of death.

Study after study has demonstrated the inability of political science to seriously link disease with tobacco, except perhaps the demonstration of an increased statistical risk of lung cancer. The dogma from which political science has proceeded in the last 30 years (tobacco IS the cause of disease) continues to lack credibility. Nevertheless, hundreds of millions of dollars keep pouring into the coffers of the anti-tobacco-environmentalist lobby to crush Demon Tobacco.

It is quite possible that the use of tobacco will be greatly reduced, at least in North America, but "the rule of unintended consequences" may come into play:

The light-to-moderate smokers, those who are not addicted to tobacco, may be induced to give up smoking "for the good of their health and the health of the nation." That's a strong message to one who smokes casually but can take it or leave it. The unintended consequence is that this group is the one <u>specifically benefiting</u> from smoking. Their health will be possibly compromised by not getting small doses of nicotine on a regular basis. The addicted smoker will continue on his destructive path to the pulmonary ward of the hospital.

Ref: Demonstration of Chlamydia pneumoniae in the walls of abdominal aortic aneurisms. Journal of Vascular Surgery, Mar 1997.

Prospective relations between Helicobacter pylori infection, coronary heart disease, and stroke in middle-aged men, Heart, Mar. 1996.

Smoking and the Decline in Heart Attack Deaths

As the anti-smoking fanatics will tell you: "It is perfectly obvious that the decrease in smoking and the decrease in death from heart disease have gone to-gether". This is indeed obvious but it does not mean that the one (decrease in smoking) caused the other (decrease in heart disease). How can there be any argument on this? Well, there can be <u>plenty</u> of argument on this.

The history of communicable diseases over the past 60 years is a good case in point. Immunization gets the credit for the dramatic decline in many communicable diseases but all of these diseases were in rapid decline long before immunizations became mandatory - polio, chicken pox, mumps, whooping cough. Malaria is an excellent example in reverse. They have never been able to produce an effective malaria vaccine. Yet, malaria has been essentially eliminated in modern communities through public health initiatives that eliminated the mosquito's breeding grounds. If there had been a "successful" vaccine produced, the vaccine would have gotten the credit.

From 1963 (the peak year) to 1985, the age-adjusted death rate fell by 42%. But the decline in ischemic heart disease (IHD) has been much greater than the decline in smoking. And when the data are analyzed by sex, the discrepancy is even more marked.

Smoking has declined less in women than in men (16% v 37%), and even anti-smokers claim less IHD risk in women from smoking, yet the decline in IHD has been proportionally equal in men and women. Women began quitting later than men, but their decline began at the same time. Said another way, while women continued to smoke, their decline in heart disease paralleled that of men who had quit smoking.

A much greater percentage of older women smoke than in the past, which would supposedly cause an increase in the death rates in those age groups, yet the decline in IHD has been about the same as at younger ages. Women's IHD death rates declined in 26 countries from 1950 to 1978, while men's death rates increased in most of those countries during this time.

Other factors that doctors like to invoke in the argument for smoking cessation don't explain the IHD decline, either. Deaths from high blood pressure began declining around 1950, while IHD was still increasing. Death rates fell just as quickly among the old, who did not embrace the exercise mania of the young (Big muscles do not equate to Big Health). IHD increased during the Depression, rather than decreasing as they would if a "rich diet" caused it. The decline began before there were any large-scale changes in diet, which are not sufficient to account for it anyhow.

Whatever caused the decline affected both sexes, and all ages and races, simultaneously and equally, with greater strength than any known influence. The 1978 Conference on the Decline in Coronary Heart Disease Mortality (of the National Heart, Blood, and Lung Institute) concluded that <u>they did not know why the rise occurred, why it ended, or why it turned downward</u>. Like other explanations, decreased smoking does not fit the paradigm.

> Mortality data are from Vital Statistics of the United States 1950-1989.
>
> Preface and Appendix in: Trends in coronary heart disease.
>
> New York: Oxford Univ Press, 1988. pp vii-x.
>
> The Rise and Fall of Ischemic Heart Disease. Sci Am 1980 Nov;243(5):53-59.
>
> Time trends for coronary heart disease mortality and morbidity. In: Trends in coronary heart disease. New York: Oxford Univ Press, 1988. pp 7-15, Ch 1.

The Monica Project

The MONICA Project was established in the early 1980s in many centers around the world to <u>MONI</u>tor trends in <u>CA</u>rdiovascular diseases and to relate these to risk-factor changes in the population over a ten year period. It was set up to explain the diverse trends in cardiovascular disease mortality, which was observed from the 1970s onwards. There are a total of 32 MONICA-collaborating Centers in 21 countries. The total population, age 25-64 years, being monitored is ten million men and women. Ten-year data collection has been completed, and most of the main results have been published.

The mere size of the study, performed by statistically minded researchers, would make the conclusions hard to ignore. But there is a major flaw in the study that I will elaborate on in a minute. In North America, the drive to ban smoking as a virtual death threat to every man, woman, and dog, is at a white-heat intensity. This study should fortify the tobaccophobics to roll up their sleeves and try harder – they have not made their case.

This monumental battle for the hearts, minds, and lungs of America is approaching the absurd. It boils down to this: The studies are meaningless. We know, and it has been known for hundreds of years, that excessive smoking is deleterious to your health. The MONICA Project, as monumental as it was, didn't prove anything not already known; it's just a monument to obfuscatory statistics.

Like alcohol, sugar and starch, excessive smoking is not good for you. The last hope for moderate smokers not to be persecuted and prosecuted for mass contamination of the universe is to convince the average, sensible citizen that side stream smoke is not a danger to the health of the people. This brilliant tactic of the anti-tobacco fanatics, completely bogus and so proven, is the atomic bomb that will fracture the nation, as did the War of Northern Aggression against the Confederate States. The legal implications alone – the loss of civil liberties of a despised minority – in itself will have severe repercussions. Who will be next? – fat people, old people, nose pickers, rich people, masturbators, gun owners, or the perfect and sanctimonious YOU?

The above paragraph is incidental I admit, as this "monumental" study did not address the issue of ETS – Environmentally Transmitted Smoke. It just condemned smoking as a political necessity. If they want to contribute something significant to the study of heart disease, they should go back to their statistics and gas chambers and honestly analyze the content, concentration and toxicity in rats of their much-hated side stream smoke. They will be disappointed and many will commit suicide - death by cigar smoke, direct - not side stream - inhalation.

"Can I have a fag and a Chip Butty Now?"

This was the headline in a British newspaper. For those of you who are not acquainted with the peculiarities of "English English," this translates into American English as: "May I have a cigarette and a sugar-coated yuk now?"

Because of the inexplicable drop in coronary artery disease in the U.S., the World Health Organization's MONICA project was commenced in the 1980s. Preliminary results were presented at the European Congress of Cardiology in Vienna in August 1998. The conclusion of the study was that all of the risk factors – obesity cholesterol, blood pressure, exercise, smoking, etc. – were significant to varying degrees.

But Hugh Tunstall-Pedoe, who was involved in the MONICA Project, says the media "metamorphosed" the original report. Some journalists claimed, on the basis of the results of the MONICA project, that coronary risk factors no longer mattered. Can you imagine the American press reporting that, even if it was true?

"The scatter plots of the 38 centers showed an unexpectedly weak relation between the size of the decline in disease rates and in individual risk factors, Dr.

Tunstall-Pedoe reported. "There were possible technical explanations," he explained. He added: "Although some centers had previously reported no change in case fatality during the revolution in treatment of myocardial infarction of the 1980s, scatter plots showed <u>an unexpectedly strong relation</u> between trends in treatment and in case fatality."

"Study casts doubt on heart 'risk factors'" was the headline in the *Daily Telegraph* on August 25th. "The largest ever cardiology study has failed to find a link between heart attacks and the classic risk factors, such as smoking and high cholesterol levels." I have always found the Telegraph to be reliable. Not that they are perfect and maybe they were as confused by Tunstall-Pedoe's report as I was.

Questions come to mind. How reliable are "scatter plots"? How can "scatter plots" show <u>an unexpectedly weak relation</u> and also an unexpectedly <u>strong relation</u>? OK, there <u>is</u> a difference in the two paragraphs below, which are verbatim from the doctor's report. (Emphasis added.)

"I drafted the press release accompanying this presentation; it emphasized the value of the data on trends collected from the 38 populations and listed findings for coronary disease rates, 28 day case fatality, smoking, blood pressure, cholesterol, and obesity. Then came the surprises. Although some centers had previously reported no change in case fatality during the revolution in treatment of myocardial infarction of the 1980s, <u>scatter plots showed an unexpectedly strong relation between trends in treatment and in case fatality</u> and also in mortality and event rates."

"Contrariwise, North Karelia and Iceland had reported (in the *BMJ*) good relations between their decline in coronary disease rates and in risk factors. The scatter plots of the 38 centers showed an unexpectedly weak relation between the size of the <u>decline in disease rates</u> and in individual risk factors, and in a composite risk factor score. There were possible technical explanations. How much the conventional risk factors might explain awaited further analyses. Meanwhile, there was room for extraneous factors that MONICA was not equipped to identify."

Why were both findings "unexpected"? Just thought I would ask.

Which is the most important, "trends in treatment" or "size of the decline in disease rates"? I vote for "decline in disease rates" and there was an "unexpectedly weak relation" between declines in disease and individual risk factors. If you are still with me, I must admit to a certain amount of confusion on my part. The whole thing seems a ball of deatomized air. I mean no disrespect to the hundreds of researchers who took part in this study, but I must agree with the Telegraph that: "The largest ever cardiology study has failed to find a link between heart attacks and the classic risk factors, such as smoking and high cholesterol levels."

The World Health Organization (WHO) has failed to make a case against the fashionable risk factors in heart disease. Even worse, the investigators ignored (in 38 languages) <u>the major suspects</u> in cardiovascular disease altogether: infection of the cardiovascular tree, folate deficiency, carbohydrate addiction, fluoride poisoning, aluminum poisoning and iron overload.

What did MONICA say? MONICA said: "Your statistics tell us nothing – start over."

To read Tunstall-Pedoe's entire article see "Monica Project" in the Appendix.

The Real Causes of Heart Disease
Help from an Unlikely Source.

While Ancel Keys' nutritional research has been proven dead wrong, his observations on tobacco and health were a landmark work that has held up under time, and mountains of propaganda. His sloppy and irresponsible research on cholesterol has been considered irrefutable by most, and has resulted in distorted, nutritional advice given to three generations of Americans. This has resulted in billions of dollars spent on the wrong food and billions more spent on cholesterol testing and anti-cholesterol drugs, not to mention more billions from taking bad advice from the gullible medical profession. Cholesterol phobia has been an unprecedented nutritional disaster.

But Key's "Seven Countries" studies of the 1960s proved that <u>smoking rates do not correlate with the wide variations in heart disease rates between different countries</u>. This astute observation does not make up for all his bad advice on cholesterol, but it helps.

There were the usual iterations about "puzzling" and "paradoxical" findings in the Keys report in that some countries had high rates of smoking but in that same country, <u>non</u>smokers had lower rates of heart disease than would be expected. In those days, no one had heard of the side stream smoke menace and so there was no mention of this. There are simple answers to this "paradox": The smokers <u>inhaled</u> but they didn't <u>exhale</u> or, side stream smoke is good for you.

"Differences in the all-causes mortality or coronary death rate or the coronary incidence rates of the cohorts could not be shown to be related to any measure of the smoking habits of the cohorts -- the proportion of the men who were nonsmokers, the proportion who were heavy smokers, the average cigarettes per day, and so on." (Seven Countries: A multivariate analysis of death and coronary heart disease, Ancel Keys, p. 325).

Well now, for the "paradox" – smokers in countries with low rates of heart disease <u>have lower rates of heart disease than non-smokers in countries with high rates</u>. Does that mean that everybody should be smoking? Does that mean that smokers are killing all those around them while they themselves stand tall? That's a little confusing but we can make it more so: Do nonsmokers in countries with low rates of heart disease have more, less, or the same rate of heart disease as smokers? The bottom line is: <u>there is no plausible relationship between smoking and heart disease</u>.

It is highly unlikely that obesity, lack of exercise, cholesterol, stress, or cigarette smoke – side stream or front stream – cause heart disease. There are many factors associated with heart disease that the doctors have only reluctantly accepted as etiologic in cardiovascular disease: homocysteine (took 25 years), excess tissue iron levels (still struggling for recognition), folate deficiency (now accepted), fluoride poisoning from water (never will be accepted), and vegetarian-like, high sugar, high starch diets (perhaps will be when the present generation of wrongheaded dieticians, cardiologists and politicians who devastated our health in the 20th Century die off from heart disease and cancer.)

The latest finding on etiology of heart disease is related to microbiology – bacterial and possibly viral involvement in the process of atherosclerosis. The evidence is overwhelming and it cannot be ignored. But the anti-tobacco scientists have an answer: "It may be a <u>cofactor</u> with tobacco." But tobacco has become the main culprit in atherosclerosis and it must remain so. This is essential to the cause, that is, their own survival, in view of recent revelations that the diet they have been recommending for 50 years is <u>the main cause</u> of hardening of the arteries. And the cofactors, if there are any, may be all the agents mentioned above: homocysteine, iron excess, folate deficiency, fluoride – and, yes, nicotine used in excess.

It is important to know a little about the infection, homocysteine and other risk factors for hardening of the arteries because <u>smoking is taking the heat for all of them</u>.

Homocysteine is a good example of this "blame-it-on-tobacco" approach. An article in Lancet is typical of this bias. It was found that <u>heart disease does correlate with elevated homocysteine levels</u>. (*Plasma homocysteine and cardiovascular disease mortality*. The Lancet Feb 1997.) When confronted with these findings from an important medical journal, the response is: "Homocysteine might play perhaps as large a role as smoking," (Newsweek 1997 August 11, "The Heart Attackers," by Geoffrey Cowley). You get the picture – there may be other factors but smoking is Number One in causation of practically every disease in W.A.D. Anderson's Textbook of Pathology.

Howard gave the appearance of trying his best to exonerate tobacco smoke in his study. He said: "We threw everything but the kitchen sink at the data but it didn't change anything." This was <u>histrionics</u>, also known as blowing smoke, and was not even close to the truth. The truth is, Howard and his associates manipulated their study groups to come to their conclusions on the influence of side stream smoke on disease.

The tobaccophobics also blamed peptic ulcer and gastritis on smoking. This came back to haunt them when a medical student discovered that peptic ulcer was cause by a bacterium – Helicobacter pylori. The same backfire may happen with the "smoking heart," but this backfire, if the truth gets out, will be heard around the world. Chlamydia pneumoniae and other microorganisms have been shown to play a part in atherosclerosis. Some critics of the findings say the organisms are just "opportunistic," meaning they move in when the arteries get sick. That's what they said about peptic ulcers, until a medical student proved they had been in error ("hyperacidity" causes peptic ulcer) for 100 years.

There is an interesting aside to the peptic ulcer-infection connection in that the experts tried to blame smoking for peptic ulcer. The American Heart Association, those scientific pretenders who claim to speak for all cardiologists, proclaimed: "This study (by Howard) provides more evidence that in order to protect the health of all non-smokers, particularly children, smoking must be banned in all public places, including restaurants"

Now let's look at the truth and see what really should be banned. The main vector of H. Pylori infection is a child, between the ages of seven and 13. The children bring the infection home to the adults from their school. This indicates that, rather than smokers causing ulcers and heart disease in children, children cause ulcers and heart disease in adults. The most important public health measure would not be banning smoking in public places but inducing children to wash their hands and keep their fingers out of their noses. If you have children you know this is not likely to happen. So perhaps we should ban children "…in

all public places, including restaurants." – at least until their H. pylori is cleared up.

The only truthful statement Howard made is that
the magnitude of their claimed ETS risk is "unbelievable." It certainly is unbelievable, and informed people
find it far more credible that the damage is due to the
risk factors they left out of the study, not to side
stream smoke. But the uninformed tend to take the
word "unbelievable" as a recommendation for its credibility. By "unbelievable, " they mean the popular version of the word, as in: "Their victory was
unbelievable." i.e., amazing. So let's straighten this
out. Their findings were indeed unbelievable, in that
they are <u>not to be believed</u>. Do I make myself clear? If
Howard had thrown the kitchen sink at the data, the
data would not have proven what he claimed to prove.
It only proved that some scientists are as gullible as
their readers.

The American Heart Association chimed in: "`<u>If a
non-smoker is around a person who smokes a pack of
cigarettes during the day, the non-smoker's exposure
is so great that it's almost comparable to his or her
smoking half of that pack of cigarettes.</u>" (AUBREY
TAYLOR, PH.D., an AHA spokesperson and lead author
of an American Heart Association statement on environmental tobacco smoke) This preposterous statement is actually believed by millions of Americans. It
has created a national panic and extreme hostility toward smokers because they, in their brainwashed, fe-
vered minds, are certain smokers are killing our
children, poisoning everyone with carbon monoxide,
causing stroke and peptic ulcers and they are destroy-
ing Medicare. Smokers are causing insanity, ear infections, asthma, miscarriages, birth defects, impotence,
and – of course – emphysema and cancer. If this is

true, then smokers are <u>the greatest danger the American people have ever faced</u>, far worse than Hitler, Mussolini, Stalin, Rosie O'Donnell, and the Headless Horseman. Shouldn't they all (smokers) be burned alive? (After a fair trial, of course.)

But before the burning starts please note that the study found "...there was no evidence of <u>a dose-response relationship</u> between increasing weekly hours of environmental smoke exposure and increased progression rates of disease." As I have pointed out elsewhere in this book, no one attempts to define their smoking cohort as to the <u>dosage of smoke</u> they're getting daily. Did they smoke a pack of coffin nails a day? Two packs a day, or maybe just six cigs a day? Does it make a difference? Yes, it makes a BIG difference because all these studies condemning cigarettes are INVALID without factoring in the "dose of the poison." As some ancient doctor/philosopher pointed out: **"The difference between a poison and a medicine is the dose."** By ignoring, or playing down <u>other risk factors</u> connected with smoking and ignoring the <u>dose-response requirements</u> in any biological study, the American Heart Association and other pseudo scientific (and some scientific) organizations can get away with just about anything.

The Journal of the American Medical Association placed its official seal of approval on scientific fraud: "Not much is passive about 'passive smoke,'" wrote the editorial authors, Rachel Werner and Dr. Thomas Pearson of the University of Rochester School of Medicine in Rochester, N.Y. "What is passive is our lack of recognition of the importance of passive smoke as a cardiovascular disease risk factor, our oversight in not asking patients about this exposure, and our lack of advocacy for clean air as a way to help prevent chronic disease," they wrote (Associated Press). Their indifference to <u>the real risk factors</u> and to <u>scientific integrity</u> can be characterized a lot more harshly than merely "passive," -- How about "irresponsible," "disgraceful," and "deceitful?" (Unfair too.)

See Appendix: The Real Causes of Heart Disease

Ref: Lancet February 1997.

Ref: <u>Carol Thompson</u>, Smokers' Rights Action Group P.O. Box 259575 Madison,WI.

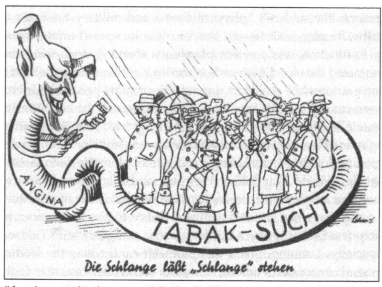

Die Schlange läßt „Schlange" stehen

"Angina and tobacco addiction". This is my favorite because it exposes those phony Nazi doctors. Most of the doctors joined the Nazi party, some out of belief in the racial cause and many out of fear. They claimed, way back in 1941, that smoking caused angina and addiction ("Tabak-Sucht") They were wrong on both counts – just like our doctors who are following their lead in misinforming the American people.

CHAPTER 2
<u>Neurological Diseases</u>

Senile Brain Disease

First in importance in the medical discoveries about tobacco is the evidence of alleviation and prevention of senile brain disease (mislabeled Alzheimer's disease).

"A statistically significant inverse relation between smoking and Alzheimer's disease was observed at all levels of analysis, with a trend towards decreasing risk with increasing consumption".

This is disturbing news to those fanatics who hate tobacco and good news for those who smoke it.

Ref: http://www.forces.org/evidence/carol/carol16.htm

Latest finding: Smoking drives you crazy, or... only crazy people smoke!

"ALMOST 50% OF ALL CIGARETTES SMOKED BY MENTALLY ILL!! BIG TOBACCO APPEARS TO BE AWARE OF THE LINK!!"

"MENTALLY ILL TWICE AS LIKELY TO BE SMOKERS, STUDY FINDS! SPECIAL PROGRAMS MAY BE NEEDED!"

Ref: Mental Disease and Tobacco Use, Los Angeles Times, 11/22/00.

Golly, it's worse than we thought. We've got to DO something about Big Tobacco – they're driving us all <u>crazy</u>, to say nothing of the rotten teeth, heart disease, deformed babies, and HALLITOSIS. We are in such a desperate situation that I think it's time to institute the DEATH PENALTY for anyone smoking within 500 yards of a church, hospital, government building or animal shelter. And we must prohibit absolutely all smoking in sports bars, pool halls and wrestling matches. This is where degenerate men and prostitutes like to smoke the most. We'll hit them where it hurts and wipe out smoking forever.

People who suffer from mental illnesses (like those nicotine-deficient screwballs described in the previous paragraph), according to Harvard Medical School research, smoke nearly half of all cigarettes purchased in the United States. Harvard "research" sounds more like a product of Stalin's *Pavlov Institute* rather than a respected medical school, at least when they abandon science for sociology as they have with the smoking issue.

And that minority medical organization, the American Medical Association, that claims to speak for all doctors, sounds more like Hitler's *Der Sturmer* with every successive issue of its journal. They have pilled on with the pinko propagandists at Harvard by publishing their preposterous polemic on "smoking drives you crazy," or "only crazy people smoke." The AMA has been after your guns and now they want your brain.

"Mentally ill people are roughly twice as likely to smoke cigarettes as those without mental illnesses," according to the research, published in the Journal of the American Medical Association, 11/22/00. "Not only does the habit put them at greater risk for serious ailments such as heart disease and lung cancer, but in some cases it can interfere with the effectiveness of medications to treat their disorders" reports Rosie Mestel of the LA Times.

Mestel continues: "Smoking is often used as a form of self-medication because nicotine can have a powerful impact on mood, according to previous research. And because people with mental illnesses tend to be more cut off from mainstream society and less able to motivate themselves to quit, it may take specially targeted educational efforts to reduce the smoking rates in this group, experts say." I don't suppose the Big Brains from Harvard ever considered the idea that the mentally ill smoke because <u>it relieves their symptoms</u>. Apparently it is OK for Big Pharma to dose them with brain-depressing drugs but it is <u>not</u> OK for them to smoke the herb, tobacco, and thus feel better while remaining alert rather than depressed from Thorazine.

"What works on ordinary, mentally healthy adults may not work as well when we're dealing with adults with mental problems," said John Banzhaf, executive director of Action on Smoking and Health, a Washington-based nonprofit advocacy group and a professor of public interest law at George Washington University. Mestel is just reporting what these "experts" tell her, but do you think there is any chance that a guy in this position – "Executive Director of Action on Smoking & Health" -- and a lawyer-professor to boot, is going to be unbiased? Well, John, let me give you my very biased opinion of your opinion: What works on "ordinary, mentally healthy adults" may not work as well on lawyer-professors with an axe to grind. If you read all the research on the issue of smoking and mental disease, you would know that tobacco smoke, <u>in moderate amounts</u>, is clearly of benefit to many mentally disturbed or brain-damaged patients, such as senile brain disease.

"The researchers found that a person who had suffered from a mental illness during the month before the interview, or at some time in the past, was more likely to smoke or have smoked in the past. In fact, those who reported a mental illness during the prior month were nearly three times as likely to be current smokers as those who didn't have a mental illness," reports Mestel. So what does that mean? It means that people with mental problems (however you define it) may get benefit from smoking because it relieves their symptoms.

From the survey, the scientists estimated that 44.3% of the cigarettes smoked in the United States are smoked by the mentally ill. That is a preposterous statement on its face. It implies that cigarettes drove them crazy. I <u>know</u> it doesn't exactly <u>say</u> that, but I know how the common man thinks, since I am one.

"The link between other mental illnesses and cigarette smoking is also well known," says Dr. Ernest Noble, Professor of Psychiatry at UCLA. "Patients smoke to enhance mood: thus, not illogically, antidepressants have been found to help people quit smoking. And in the case of schizophrenia, the medications that patients must take alter chemicals in their brains, causing a despondency that smoking alleviates," says Noble.

Now, Rosie, I know you are not a psychopharmical psychiatrist so I assume Dr. Noble gave you these pharmacological insights into the inner workings of these magical drugs. But let me ask, and perhaps Dr. Noble can give you an answer, if the medication causes despondency, why are they taking it in the first place? They are taking these mind-altering drugs <u>for the benefit of the doctors and the staff</u> to make the patients more malleable. They do nothing positive for the patient. A deluded patient may come in thinking he's a king and he is quickly turned into a cabbage. These mind-altering drugs are clearly therapeutic – but for the staff and not the patient.

If smoking is "linked" to mental illness, as Dr. Noble claims, ask him to show you sound scientific evidence to back up that assertion. And one more question: If smoking alleviates the patient's despondency, caused by "altering chemicals in their brains," why shouldn't they smoke?

"Some studies suggest," Rosie continues, "that certain mental illnesses may be triggered or exacerbated by smoking, again perhaps because of its mood-altering potential. For instance, in an article in the Journal of the American Medical Association, published earlier this month, scientists reported that adolescents and young people who smoked heavily were more likely to develop anxiety disorders later in life." Are these young people suffering from anxiety because they smoke or do they smoke to relieve their anxiety? What is worse, taking dangerous mind-altering drugs or smoking a few stogies a day?

"People who suffer from mental illnesses are also more likely to be poor -- and smoking is strongly linked to poverty," says our friend Professor John Banzhaf, executive director of Action on Smoking and Health. "And quitting cigarettes requires long-term planning, impulse control and the ability to personalize risk -- all that much harder to do when one's thinking is impaired by mental illness." [Or impaired by drugs?]

I wonder how Banzhaf will initiate his "impulse control" treatment. Mandatory electric shock therapy should be very effective (in the short run).

Are the povert's poor because they smoke or do they smoke to relieve the depression and anxiety of being poor? Which is the cheaper for the poor povert – a few cigs or cigars per day or the institutionalization of the patient and the use of incredibly expensive drugs? Well why worry? The (smoking) taxpayers will pay the bill through ruthless taxation of cigarettes and cigars, the medical staff makes good money and the drug industry gets bigger and richer.

The authors of the latest paper also suggest that the tobacco industry may have been aware of the "psychological vulnerability" of part of their market. The scientists quote a 1981 document by R.J. Reynolds Tobacco Co., which noted that some smokers smoked for "mood enhancement" and "positive stimulation" or because smoking "helps perk you up," "calm down," and "cope with stress," says Mestel. <u>Horrors</u>!

That sounds like a pretty good herb to me. You can <u>keep</u> your potent pills from the big dope pharm. I'd rather cope with my "psychological vulnerability" with a nice, aromatic, Nicaraguan robusto cigar.

There are other innuendoes in this article. In summary:

- Smoking drives you crazy.
- Mostly crazy people smoke.
- Smoking causes poverty.
- Smoking interferes with the action of the mind-altering drugs used against mental disease. (And that is a good thing).
- Smoking causes cardiovascular disease.

- Smoking causes lung cancer. (If done in excess, probably true.)

Light up; don't over do it; be happy – and stay away from psychiatrists!

See Appendix: Smoking and Schizophrenia by Norman Swan.

Ref: ROSIE MESTEL, Los Angeles Times, 11/22/00.

American Journal of Epidemiology, Vol 147, Issue 12.

Alzheimer's

This disease, like Parkinson's disease, is an insidious killer and robber of life. People with AD have a considerably decreased life expectancy with the course of the disease taking away an average of 8 years. AD is a specific combination of brain features that include loss of certain areas of the brain and damaging plaques and tangles of the wires of the brain. It is difficult sometimes to distinguish this disease from others because of other forms of dementias that may be present so as many as 80% of AD cases can go unrecognized by doctors.

It is important to note that we are referring to "pre-senile dementia," NOT senile brain deterioration, as in the case of President Reagan. AD has an onset early in life – in the 40s or 50s. Even some doctors are confused on this diagnosis. However, it may be that nicotine has benefit in <u>both</u> conditions.

It has been discovered that acute administration of low doses of nicotine <u>improved</u> mental processes and may be protective in AD. There is a clear negative association between smoking and AD. Not only is there a clear negative association but also studies have found that nicotine improves attention and information processing in patients with AD.

One study states:

"The risk of Alzheimer's disease decreased with increasing daily number of cigarettes smoked before onset of disease. In six families in which the disease was apparently inherited, the mean age of onset was 4-17 years later in smoking patients than in non-smoking from the same family." (Conelia M. van Duljn MSC, Albert Hoffman Md., Erasmus University Medical School).

To see a complete list of studies and publications on tobacco and Alzheimer's and Parkinson's disease see Appendix: Alzheimer's and Parkinson's disease.

Ref: http://www.forces.org/evidence/files/liars.htm#alz

Parkinson's

The neurological disease most dreaded by the elderly after Alzheimer's is Parkinson's. As with Alzheimer's, modern medicine has no satisfactory treatment for senile brain degeneration. A long-term study found an inverse association of smoking dose and Parkinson's disease.

A study titled "Twin Study Supports Protective Effect of Smoking For Parkinson's disease" by the Tanner Group did retrospective studies going back 20 years. They concluded that smoking in the early years and then quitting, still had a positive effect in preventing Parkinson's. And the longer you smoke, the less likely you are to get PD. "'The inverse association of smoking dose and PD can be attributed to environmental, and not genetic causes with near certainty," the authors write.

There has been a total silence from the anti-smoking mass media on this pivotal, long-range study that shows yet another benefit of smoking. If the intention of "public health" is to inform the public about the consequences of smoking on health as it proclaims, why don't we see "warnings" such as:

"Smoking Protects Against Parkinson's Disease!,"

or

"Smoking Protects Against Alzheimer's Disease!,"

or

"Smoking Protects Against Ulcerative Colitis!"

And so on, alongside with the other speculations on "tobacco-related" disease? Isn't the function of public health to tell the citizens about ALL the effects on health of a substance? "Public Health," today, is nothing more than a deceiving propaganda machine paid by pharmaceutical and public money to promote frauds, fears, and puritanical rhetoric dressed up in white coats.

The bibliography of references offered in this book should convince the most passionate of anti-smokers that if you <u>don't</u> smoke then you could run the risk of getting Parkinson's Disease or Alzheimer's. But the anti-smoking groups, backed by several medical journals (more interested in advertising revenue than in informing the population), are silent. *It could be reasonably asserted that non-smokers are a burden to society due to their tendency to contract these diseases.* Therefore, because they didn't smoke during their young and middle years, they led a long and useless old age, a burden to themselves and their families.

See Appendix: Twin Study Supports Protective Effect of Smoking For Parkinson's disease.

Ref: http://www.forces.org

Ref: Reuters Medical News March 5, 2002 http://193.78.190.200/10m/twin.htm

Tourette's

If we are going to discuss the treatment of Tourette's syndrome with nicotine, then you should know what it is. It's a bizarre disease, to put it mildly. It is characterized by strange behavior, both vocal and physical. This is characterized by uncontrollable, sudden outbursts: "Yap," the patient may expostulate vigorously, and then continue his conversation as if nothing had happened. It is both amusing and tragic. Children will laugh, thinking the person is entertaining them. Unfortunately, their outbursts are often vulgar and salacious: "F... your mother!" Obviously, this is acutely embarrassing to all concerned, especially the patient, if he is aware of it, and they often are. Suicide is not uncommon. Physically, there may be a sudden writhing of the head, as if the patient was strangling, but it then goes away. Cigar smoking should be tried where practicable. If the condition is severe to the point of making life in a polite society impossible, intravenous nicotine should be tried.

The University of South Florida did a milestone study on the effects of tobacco and people with Tourette's syndrome. Although nicotine patches are a crude method of delivery, compared to smoking cigars, smoking a water pipe, or using intravenous nicotine drip injections, their results were astounding. The King TV Seattle report said the researchers found that the nicotine patches "boosted the effectiveness of drugs given" to relieve Tourette's symptoms. We suspect that the results of the nicotine therapy might have been <u>even better</u> without the use of the drugs.

They followed patients ranging in age from nine to 15 who responded poorly to haloperidol (Haldol) or other drugs commonly given to treat Tourette's. NONE of these drugs are effective in doing <u>anything</u> but depressing the patient. If you depress the patient you may have the warm feeling that you are treating their <u>disease</u>, but the therapist is only treating <u>himself</u>. When the drug was combined with a low dose nicotine patch, the "benefits of the medication" increased an average of 45 percent. Patients wore the patch for 24 hours and then removed it. Relief from symptoms occurred within three hours of administering the patch <u>and was maintained up to 10 days after the patch was removed</u>.

We must emphasize: The results would probably be better without the depressing effect of drugs that are used to "treat" practically anything, from Tourette's to shop-lifting. In fact, patients given a choice invariably choose the nicotine treatment over the antipsychotic drugs, Dr. Paul R. Sanberg, professor and chair of neuroscience at the University of South Florida, reported. The drugs have potent and extremely unpleasant side effects. The only side effect of the nicotine is an improvement in the condition.

As you might expect, such an effective chemical shows great promise in the treatment of other neurological and undefined "nervous" disorders, such as ADHD. The exceptionally high rates of smoking among people afflicted with Attention Deficit Hyperactivity Disorder (ADHD), depression and schizophrenia suggest that nicotine might provide some relief. Studies have already shown an improvement in cognitive ability among schizophrenics and a greater ability to focus among ADHD patients who wear a nicotine patch.

I have been asked: "Do you expect <u>children</u> to smoke cigars, or a water pipe, or – God help us – cigarettes?" My answer is that God has already "helped us" by creating the sacred (to me anyway) tobacco plant. He gave us the power to reason and to overcome our prejudices based on false science and government propaganda. I don't care <u>how</u> the children get the nicotine if they are nicotine-deficient, as many of them appear to be, so long as they get it. I have a compromise between the not-maximally-effective nicotine patch and the spectacle of a six-year-old puffing on a cigar – sublingual nicotine lozenges or oral tablets. I don't know if either of these have been investigated, but they should be.

See Appendix:
- Nicotine: helping those who help themselves? By John A. Rosecrans.
- A Cigarette Chemical Packed With Helpful Effects? By John Schwartz.
- News Anchor reports on USF study. By Julie Francavilla.
- Nicotine for the Treatment of Tourette's syndrome.

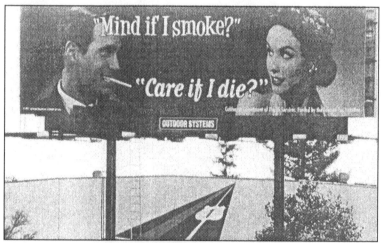

In private, they usually say it in a more vulgar way. But how can anyone believe such a preposterous lie in the first place? – but millions do.

CHAPTER 3
Women, Children and Tobacco

A Stogie A Day Keeps Eclampsia Away!

As with the "smoking-causes-miscarriage" issue, the truth with tobacco and eclampsia is the opposite of popular opinion. Again, junk science rules popular thought.

Preeclampsia is primarily a disease of the last trimester of pregnancy although symptoms may appear earlier. It is characterized by high blood pressure, protein in the urine, headaches, blurring of vision and seizures. It can be deadly. Liver and kidney damage are the major serious complications of eclampsia, also known as "toxemia of pregnancy." The fetus can be severely damaged.

A study from the University of Pittsburgh, found that "While smoking during pregnancy has many adverse health effects on mother and fetus, it appears to decrease the risk of preeclampsia." -- Kristine Yoder Lain, assistant professor of obstetrics, gynecology and reproductive sciences at the University of Pittsburgh School of Medicine. Well, Christine, if you had your pregnant patients smoke three cigars a day, you would find that there would not be "many adverse health effects on mother and fetus." In fact...there wouldn't be ANY adverse effects. And while training your patients to smoke stogies, you might light up yourself.

OK, cigar lovers, there's the answer you've been waiting for: <u>Smoking during pregnancy reduces the risk of eclampsia and many other conditions related to pregnancy</u>. So light up, Little Mother, and smoke yourself to a safe delivery and a healthy baby. And you, Daddy, can get ready to pass out the cigars. (I <u>love</u> this job!)

See Appendix: Is Smoking Bad for Eclampsia Patients.

Ref: Am J Obstet Gynecol 1999;181 University Times (University of Pittsburgh), Volume 34, Number 20, June 13, 2002.

Does Maternal Smoking Hinder Mother-Child Transmission of Helicobacter Pylori Infection?

"Everybody knows" that a mother should not smoke during pregnancy. Smoking during pregnancy, or even being in a room with smokers, is tantamount to child abuse. I wouldn't be surprised if a law were passed making it a felony for a woman to smoke during pregnancy. But is smoking during pregnancy, even in moderation, all that bad?

Helicobacter pylori is the germ that causes peptic ulcer and it may cause other mischief as well. In the research quoted below, the investigators went under the supposition that <u>mother-child transmission</u> of the bug during the preschool years was responsible for infection in the child and consequent high risk for peptic ulcer later in life.

Following is a truncated version of their summary. Their argument is quite compelling for a benefit to young children of exposure to cigarette or cigar smoke, at least regarding protection from peptic ulcer.

"Evidence for early childhood as the critical period of Helicobacter pylori infection and for clustering of the infection within families suggests a major role of interfamilial transmission. In a previous study, we found a strong inverse relation between maternal smoking and H. pylori infection among preschool children, <u>suggesting the possibility that mother-child transmission of the infection may be less efficient if the mother smokes.</u>

To evaluate this hypothesis further, we carried out a subsequent population-based study in which H. pylori infection was measured by 13C-urea breath test in 947 preschool children and their mother. We obtained detailed information on potential risk factors for infection, including maternal smoking, by standardized questionnaires. Overall, 9.8% (93 of 947 of the children and 34.7% (329 of 947) of the mothers were infected. Prevalence of infection was much lower among children of uninfected mothers (1.9%) than among children of infected mothers (24.7%). <u>There was a strong inverse relation of children's infection with maternal smoking</u> (adjusted odds ratio = infected mothers, but not among children of uninfected mothers. These results support the hypothesis of a predominant role for mother-child transmission of H. pylori infection, <u>which may be less efficient if the mother smokes.</u>" (underline added)

Ref: http://www.ncbi.nlm.nih.gov/htbin-post/Entrez/ query?uid=10615847&form=6&db=m&Dopt=b

For more information on smoking and pregnancy, see: http:// www.forces.org/evidence/evid/preg.htm>

Does Tobacco Smoke Prevent Atopic Disorders and Asthma?

If there is one thing certain, it's that women should not smoke during pregnancy - right? Let's look at the scientific truth and not the pseudo science that has led doctors to forbid an herb during pregnancy that can actually be protective to the baby. That herb is tobacco.

"In a multivariate analysis, children of mothers who smoked at least 15 cigarettes a day tended to have lower odds for suffering from allergic rhino-conjunctivitis, allergic asthma, atopic eczema and food allergy, compared to children of mothers who had never smoked. Children of fathers who had smoked at least 15 cigarettes a day had a similar tendency."

Ref: "Does tobacco smoke prevent atopic disorders? A study of two generations of Swedish residents".
http://193.78.190.200/30/asthma.htm

Children of smokers have a LOWER incidence of asthma! You certainly won't see this one on the health news of BBC or ABC, as they are too busy trying to convince us that smokers "cause" asthma in their kids - and in the kids of other people. That's not true, as smoking does not "cause" asthma. More of the smoker's paradox: <u>Smoking does not cause asthma; it may aid in the prevention of asthma.</u>

Smoking parents cause asthma in their kids and the children of others? Au contraire, my misdirected and bamboozled reader, the offspring of smokers have <u>lower</u> rates of asthma!

Effects of Transdermal Nicotine on Cognitive Performance in Down's Syndrome.

Another "paradoxical" finding has to do with Down's syndrome. Those who are totally committed to the belief that tobacco is bad in every respect and has no therapeutic use whatsoever, call the reports herein "paradoxical." An analogy would be "The antibiotic made the infection worse." Or "The more fat he ate the skinnier he got." It just isn't possible that tobacco smoke could have a beneficial effect on ANY disease. Everyone knows that to be true. Well, it ISN'T true and here is another example of an effective treatment of an incurable disease.

"We investigated the effect of nicotine-agonistic stimulation with 5 mg transdermal patches, compared with placebo, on cognitive performance (in plain English: thinking ability) in five adults with the disorder. Improvements possibly related to attention and information processing was seen for Down's syndrome patients compared with healthy controls. Our preliminary findings are encouraging…" the doctors reported.
Ref: http://193.78.190.200/13/tlj.htm

What these researchers didn't suggest, and perhaps didn't think of, is that the mucous membranes of the mouth are far more efficient in absorbing medication, such as nicotine, than the skin - at least ten times more efficient than the patch they used on the above mentioned patients. Even though it is obviously true that the Down's syndrome patients were positively affected, that would be an unsafe course for any institutional researcher to navigate. It should be noted that this was a very small study (5 cases) and so is not conclusive.

So <u>more</u> benefits of nicotine. Of course, it is politically <u>incorrect</u> to say that this is a benefit of SMOKING, it's only a positive outcome and politically CORRECT coming from the "pharmaceutically - produced" transdermal nicotine patch. They would like to imply that the nicotine that is delivered through cigarettes is terribly addictive, but when delivered through patches, it is not, and is actually beneficial! Antismoking <u>nonsense</u> aside, nicotine gets into the body regardless of the means of delivery. And more evidence about the benefits of smoking is emerging. Though the small size of this study cannot be taken as conclusive it is encouraging to smokers.

Junk Science Presses the Attack

...against smoking. You'd think, after all the huffing and puffing for the past 20 years, they would declare victory and find another "Enemy of Mankind", this time something constructive, such as anti-fluoridation. It's ironic that these phony environmentalists look the other way when you mention fluoridated water – <u>the most malignant pollution of all time</u>. And why aren't they attacking Coca Cola and all the other slimy people in the junk beverage industry? Why is that? Tobacco, especially in the form of cigars or a water pipe, has a myriad of health benefits. Can you say that about Coke or fluoride? You might hesitate to decry fluoride, since your dentist says it is good for your children. But don't fall for that propaganda disguised as science.

And now back to the latest psych-war attack against tobacco. These MDs and PhDs set out to determine if certain "risk factors" – smoking, alcohol, caffeine and "psycho-social stress," were related to an increase in attention deficit disorder and hyperactivity.

Does it take 36 studies and 11 MDs, PhDs, and PDQs to make an inconclusive conclusion? The whole thing is worthy of a Woody Allen parody, a farrago of mealy-mouth elocutions and garrulous puffballs containing nothing but innuendoes and inanities. As I chortled through this scientific chafe, I happened to glance at the name of the publication honoring these science heads from la-la land: the <u>*American Journal of Psychiatry*</u>. Oh well then, I suppose I shouldn't get so worked up about this science parody by the psycho-med crowd who don't seem to know anything worth knowing.

BUT, people think they are <u>real scientists</u> and since most of the readers are reading a reporter's interpretation of the study – and he knows little about science and medicine himself -- they believe these "scientists" are giving them the real thing – like Coca Cola.

To cover themselves, the authors discuss in the body of the report the mass of contradictions that make the survey meaningless. First, they say, "<u>A narrative approach was used</u> because the studies <u>differed too much in methods and data sources to permit a quantitative meta-analysis</u>. Putting aside the simple truth that meta-analysis epidemiological surveys are worthless (except for propaganda purposes), they admit the hopelessness of their endeavor when they state that all the studies differed in method and data sources. So, since the whole thing was a confused mess, "a narrative approach was used" which means they abandoned the scientific method all together, as in: "Can we talk?" That may be science over there in the coo coo bin but it's not science in the Department of Epidemiology, Stanford University Medical School, or any other medical school.

Clearly, the study was aimed at tobacco although they pretended to be interested in other risk factors. They looked at 24 tobacco studies and only 15 studies concerning the three other "risk factors" combined. They came to the conclusion that "in spite of inconsistencies," the studies on nicotine "indicated" a greater risk of ADHD-related disorders among children whose mothers smoked during pregnancy. Then they went on to make perfect asses of themselves by stating: "Many studies suffered from methodological shortcomings, such as recall bias, crude or inaccurate exposure assessments, low statistical power, and lack of or insufficient control of confounders. A general lack of information on familial psychopathology also limited the interpretations."

BUT, after admitting the whole thing is crapola, they say: "Exposure to tobacco smoke in utero "is suspected" to be associated with Attention Deficit Hyperactivity Disorder (ADHD) and ADHD symptoms in children." One thing psychiatrists learn in medical school is that they can sound like doctors even though they never practice medicine. Put in simple English, they are saying that if a mother smokes during her pregnancy there is an increased risk of her baby becoming a hyperactive child.

Let me add that I am not saying a mother should smoke during her pregnancy. But I am saying there is no proof that it does any harm. The mother of my children smoked two packs a day of Marlboros and she had two perfectly normal babies. I will also tell you they were raised in a cloud of cigar smoke (mine) and they are still normal. The science presented in this book is incontrovertible: <u>Moderate smoking prevents many diseases.</u>

I've changed my mind. Mother's <u>should</u> smoke during pregnancy - one stogie after lunch and one after dinner. Do not inhale. Added benefit - your constipation will be cured.

See Appendix: Junk Science Presses the Attack.

Ref: American Journal of Psychiatry 160:1028-1040, June 2003.

Maternal Smoking & Congenital Defects

The evidence is overwhelming that smoking does not cause congenital defects, either neurological or physical. Let's look at the compilation of research by Wanda Hamilton. (Underlining added)

Many studies have indicated a <u>slight decrease</u> in the rates of congenital defects for infants of smoking mothers. For example, study after study has shown that the risks of having an infant with Down's syndrome are lower for smoking mothers. "<u>There was no evidence of an association between any congenital defect and smoking</u>" is the conclusion of McDonald and his associates.

Ref: McDonald AD, et al "Cigarette, alcohol, and coffee consumption and congenital defects," American Journal of Public Health, Jan l992.

Malloy and associates " ...<u>found no increased risk (of congenital malformations) for infants of smokers.</u>" "When adjusted for potential confounders the odds ratio for congenital malformation in the infants of women who smoked during pregnancy was not increased." In fact there was <u>a slightly lower risk</u> for infants of smoking mothers.

Ref: Malloy MH, et al "Maternal smoking during pregnancy: no association with congenital malformations in Missouri 1980-83," American Journal of Public Health, Sep l989.

"<u>Neither maternal nor paternal smoking habits were significantly associated with the occurrence of congenital malformations</u>." This study involved 17,152 infants. Maternal smoking habits in 67,609 singleton pregnancies were examined. The overall incidence of congenital malformations was 2.8% in both non-smokers and smokers. On analyzing congenital defects according to individual systems there was no significant difference in the incidence of malformations according to the number of cigarettes smoked, except for neural tube defects. This study suggests that maternal smoking does not have teratogenic effects in the offspring, except in the case of neural tube defects, where the effect is at most modest."

Ref: Seidman DS, et al Obstetrics and Gynecology, Dec I990.

"<u>Parental smoking was not associated with increased risks for neural tube defects</u>."

Ref: Evans DR, et al British Medical Journal, Jul 21 I979.

"Statistically significant <u>negative associations</u> were found for ventricular septal defects, hydroceles, clubfoot, pigmented nevi, hemangiomas, and Down syndrome. For all these congenital defects, the risks were <u>significantly lower</u> for the offspring of smoking mothers."

Ref: Wasserman et al, "Parental cigarette smoking and risk for congenital anomalies of the heart, neural tube, or limb," Teratology, Apr I996.

"Based on this large series of cases, maternal smoking during pregnancy does not appear to increase the risk of oral clefts."

Ref: Shiono PH, et al "Congenital malformations and maternal smoking during pregnancy," Teratology, Aug I986.

"<u>We did not find any association with Down's syndrome or any other malformation</u>."

Ref: Werler MM, et al "Maternal cigarette smoking during pregnancy in relation to oral clefts," Am J. Epidemiol, Nov. I990.

"Collectively, our results provide <u>no evidence</u> for an association between fetal Down's syndrome and smoking. Other published studies found <u>a deficit of smokers among women who had pregnancies associated with Down's syndrome</u>."

Ref: Van den Eeden, et al "A case-control study of maternal smoking and congenital malformations," Pediatrics, Perinatology & Epidemiology, Apr l990.

"The risk of cardiovascular malformations was not associated with maternal smoking."

Ref: Cuckle et al "Maternal smoking habits and Down's syndrome," Prenatal Diagnosis Sep. l990.

"<u>No statistically significant differences</u> were found in the frequencies of CAs [chromosome aberrations] between non-smoking mothers and smoking mothers."

Ref: Tikkanen J, et al "Maternal exposure to chemical and physical factors during pregnancy and cardiovascular malformations in the offspring," Teratology, Jun l991.

"<u>No effect</u> of maternal smoking in early pregnancy observed on chromosome aberrations in chorionic villus samples."

Ref: Salonen K, et al Mutation Research, Feb l993.

The above articles appeared in nine different medical journals involving dozens of researchers. There is no equivocation in their conclusions. But who reads Mutation Research, Teratology, and Prenatal Diagnosis? However, how can the tobaccophobics ignore the British Medical Journal, the American Journal of Epidemiology, and the American Journal of Public Health? The latter journal is particularly adamant and vociferous on the subject of side stream smoke and smoking in general.

Maternal Smoking, Body Mass Index, and Neural Tube Defects

Swedish researchers have <u>more</u> surprising news for pregnant women who smoke. While the anti-smoking science apparatchiki continues their sneak-attack methods – we are now told that smoking causes hyperactivity and attention deficit disorder in children, but <u>WE</u> continue to come across articles that prove the health advantages of moderate smoking for these conditions. <u>Now</u> consider the claim that smoking during pregnancy causes neural tube defects.

The Swedish health registries were used to investigate a possible effect on the incidence of neural tube defects (NTDs) of maternal smoking and maternal body mass index (BMI) ($kg/m2$). Among 1,199,701 infants born in 1983-1993 with known smoking exposure in early pregnancy, 621 infants with NTDs were selected. After controlling for year of birth, maternal age, parity (Number of pregnancies), education level, BMI, and immigrant status (yes/no), <u>a highly significant, protective effect of maternal smoking on the incidence of NTDs was found</u>. A protective <u>dose-response effect</u> of smoking was indicated <u>but was not statistically significant</u>.

The association between NTDs and maternal body mass index (BMI) found in earlier studies was supported. Women with BMI >26.0 were found to be at higher risk of having an infant with NTD compared with women in other BMI classes. No obvious explanation was found, either for the detected association between NTDs and BMI, or for the protective effect of maternal smoking.

Scientists generally go into these studies with a strong bias against tobacco and expect to find evidence that corroborates their prejudices. So imagine the consternation among the tobacco haters when it was announced: "...<u>a highly significant, protective effect</u> of maternal smoking on the incidence of NTDs was found."

Don't be misled by the apparent contradiction in this report. <u>A highly significant, protective effect of maternal smoking</u> was found. However, they were not able to calculate the significant <u>dose response</u>, that is, the amount of smoking required to have the protective effect, that is, how much is enough? That would be difficult to determine but at least the authors recognize the importance of this parameter.

The same cannot be said for the researchers who show an extreme prejudice against smoking in any form or any amount. Their motto is: say it often, say it loudly and don't confuse the rabble with facts they do not need to know – such as, especially such as – what is the safe dosage of nicotine? The very idea of a "safe dosage" for the evil weed is heresy to them. They demand ZERO TOLERANCE – a smoke-free America.

Ref: American Journal of Epidemiology, Vol. 147, Issue 12 1103-1111.

Ref: K. Kallen, Tornblad Institute, University of Lund, Sweden.

Musculoskeletal Birth Defects

And while we are on the subject of birth defects, the tobacco-phobics are now going after smoke for causing musculoskeletal birth defects. The research on this reveals <u>no evidence</u> of a correlation between smoking and musculoskeletal disorders. As often happens, when the tobacco lumpkins go on a crusade, it backfires in their wizened faces. From the literature, which they apparently don't read, it is obvious that there is a real possibility there is a <u>reverse correlation</u> between smoking and musculoskeletal disorders. This means, in plain English, that smoking <u>decreases</u> the likelihood of these deformities taking place during pregnancy. The following graph illustrates the lack of statistical significance in matching smokers with birth defects:

Please note in the graph below that 1.0, on the left side of the graph, means that all those studies at or below that line means no risk at all. And any dots you see above that line up to 2.0 means that the risk is inconsequential. So, out of the eleven studies, only one has a dot above the 2.0 line and it is of a magnitude that makes it also of no significance.

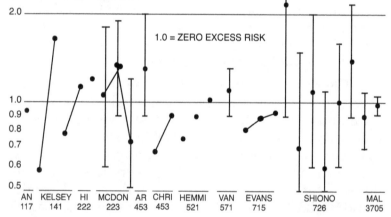

Ref: Heinonen OP, Slone D, Shapiro S, eds. **Birth defects and drugs in pregnancy.** Littleton, MA: Publishing Sciences Group, 1977. Collaborative Perinatal Project prospective. 404 musculoskeletal (including polydactyly) **smoking nonsignificance.**

Carol Thompson has done her usual excellent job of research on this non-problem and her references are listed below (Don't bother reading them; trust me, I'm a doctor!)

"Study after study fails to find ANY consistent, positive correlation between smoking and musculoskeletal birth defects. In fact, many studies show a negative correlation -- that is smoking during pregnancy could result in fewer defects than not smoking. Basically, the lack of consistency in results makes it clear that smoking is not the factor that should be under study in the matter -- it is obvious that other factors are involved." -- Courtesy of Carol Thompson Smokers' Rights Action Group. P.O. Box 259575 Madison, WI 53725-9575.

Ref: Smokers' Rights Action Group P.O. Box 259575 Madison, WI 53725-9575 Carol Thompson, 08/23/93.

Andrews J, McGarry JM. **A community study of smoking in pregnancy**. J Obstet Gynaecol Br Common: 1972 Dec; 79(12): 1057-1073.

Kelsey JL, Dwyer T, Holford TR, Bracken MB. **Maternal smoking and congenital malformations: an epidemiological study**. J Epidemiol Commun Health 1978; 32:102-107. Himmelberger DU, Brown BW, Cohen, EN. **Cigarette smoking during pregnancy and the risk of spontaneous abortion and congenital anomaly.** Am J Epidemiol 1978; 108 (6): 470-479. McDonald AD, Armstrong BG, Sloan M. **Cigarette, alcohol, and coffee consumption and congenital defects.** AJPH Jan. 1992;82(1):91-93. Aro T.

Maternal diseases, alcohol consumption and smoking during pregnancy associated with reduction limb defects. Early Human Dev. 1983;9:49-57.

Christianson RE. **The relationship between maternal smoking and the incidence of congenital anomalies.** Am J Epidemiol 1980; 112 (5):684-695. Kaiser Foundation prospective.

Hemminki K, Mutagen P, Saloniemi T: **Smoking and the occurrence on congenital malformations and spontaneous abortions: Multivariate analysis.** Am J Obstet Gynecol Jan 1 1983; 145:61-66.

Van Den Eeden SK, Karagas MR, Daling JR, Vaughan TL. **A case-control study of maternal smoking and congenital malformations.** Paediatr Perinatal Epidemiol 1990;4: 147-155.

Evans DR, Newcombe RG, Campbell H. **Maternal smoking habits and congenital malformations: a population study.** BMJ July 21 1979; 2:171-173.

Shiono PH, Klebanoff MA, Berendes HW. **Congenital malformations and maternal smoking during pregnancy.** Teratol 1986;34:65-71.

Malloy MH, Kleinman JC, Bakewell JM, Schramm WF, Land GH. **Maternal smoking during pregnancy: No association with congenital malformations in Missouri.** AJPH 1989 Sep;79(9):1243-1246.

The Big Lie - Smoking Causes Birth Defects

The obfuscation, distortion and plain lies that are used to blame smoking for every disease of man, is appalling and quite frightening as it reminds one of Nazi and Bolshevist propaganda of the 1930s.

The 1989 Surgeon General's report (*Reducing the Health Consequences of Smoking, 25 Years of Progress*) uses only two small studies in an attempt to make the case for smoking causing birth defects. But their case is NEVER made, as you will see below from <u>the studies that were **not** mentioned</u>.

The graphic below reveals the preposterousness of their claims because it clearly indicates <u>there is no correlation</u> between birth defects and smoking. Keep in mind that an excess risk factor **less than 3.0** is considered insignificant among respectable scientists. I know you don't like graphs but this one is worth your time as it reveals the deceitfulness of the Surgeon General, the fanatics in the anti-smoking industry and the holier-than-thou Puritans (and I don't mean the Pilgrims) in the science community. Who in the science industry would ever support the health benefits of tobacco?

Note in the graph below that 1.0, on the left side of the graph, means that all those studies at or below that line means no risk at all. And any dots you see above that line up to 2.0 means that the risk is inconsequential. So, out of the nine studies, none has a dot above the 2.0 line so there is no consequence.

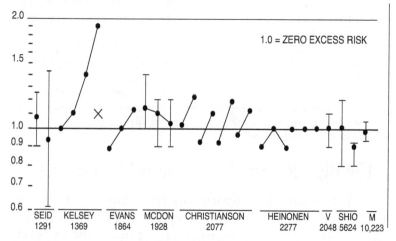

http://www.forces.org/evidence/images/cargraf1.gif

Notice the second report from the left, the Kelsey study. You will note that the risk factor is <u>less than 2.0</u> – and this is the highest of all the studies. These studies have high credibility because they all involve a large number of patients. Studies with less than a thousand cases were excluded.

"The dose makes the poison" is one of the oldest adages in medicine. Iodine, for example, is essential for thyroid health. But a large dose can kill you. That is why I have repeated the statement in this book that I am promoting **moderate** use of tobacco – even cigarettes can be harmful – if the <u>dosage</u> is incorrect. I know I will be accused of all manner of crimes for writing and publishing this book, but no amount of obfuscation can hide the fact that moderate amounts of tobacco smoke, preferably in a water pipe, or a good cigar, or a pipe is good for your health.

The dose is the thing but, in almost all of the anti-tobacco "scientific" reports, dosage is never considered. We must consider <u>the great ignored</u> parameter - the dosage of smoke and nicotine the test subjects are getting. Without this information, the studies are all just useless verbiage

The studies we are presenting <u>DO</u> consider the dosage and the response to the dose of smoke inhaled. The most remarkable revelation in these reports is that the dose, i.e., the number of cigarettes smoked and risk assumed had <u>no correlation at all</u>. In the McDonald study (MCDON on the graph), the risk of birth defects became <u>less</u> as the number of cigarettes smoked <u>increased</u>. At least in the case of maternal smoking while pregnant, there is no repeatable dose/response curve. Therefore there is no association between birth defects and smoking.

As Carol Thompson, from whom we got this excellent report said: "Using scare tactics based on misinterpretations of scientific research to change human behavior is reprehensible, irresponsible and does tremendous damage to the reputations of the vast majority of scientists who conduct careful and meticulous research."

See Appendix: Maternal Smoking References.

Ref: 1989 Surgeon General's report (Reducing the Health Consequences of Smoking, 25 Years of Progress).
Carol Thompson, 08/23/93 Smokers' Rights Action Group P.O. Box 259575 Madison, WI 53725-9575.

The California Tobacco Trashers

It isn't often that you get to discredit the tobacco trashers from their own research but the following California EPA report, "*Health Effects of Exposure to Environmental Tobacco Smoke*," is as good as it gets. The reports are supposed to have discovered the causes of perinatal and infant death. And guess what it is – ambient air ("side stream") tobacco smoke! What else?

All of their studies have a fatal (and inexcusable) investigational flaw that makes all their studies worthless and, in fact, dangerously misleading. The anti-smoking Puritans will (privately) respond that even if studies are <u>abjectly false</u>, such as these ambient air EPA reports, it's OK if they induce people to stop smoking. This is exactly what Hitler's propaganda minister, Joseph Goebels, did in his anti-smoking campaign. He got Nazi doctors, and most German doctors became Nazis, to produce reams of "studies" proving that smoking was the worst evil in the world and contrary to Arian health ideals. If you look at the cartoons in this book, you will be struck by the similarity of the Nazi cartoons of the 30s to the neo-Nazi cartoons of today. Sixty years apart, they reflect the same simplistic and childish approach that is necessary to impress the simple-minded masses. The people of the Soviet Union didn't have to suffer through all this crude propaganda – Stalin was a smoker.

So, what is the "fatal and inexcusable flaw" in the research to which I am referring? There is a condition called chorio-amnionitis that causes about 90 percent of cases of perinatal death and stillbirths. Either the placentas of the mothers in this EPA study were not tested for chorio-amnionitis or the results of the test were suppressed. But an even more likely reason would be that the investigators were completely ignorant of the disease and its importance in neonatal death and miscarriages. Resolutely armed with ignorance, the researchers could confidently proclaim "Environmental Tobacco Smoke is the major cause of miscarriages and perinatal death." Those are not their exact words but that's the message. So it matters not if the studies were fraudulent, farcical, and flatulent so long as the proper message is delivered to <u>The Great Unwashed</u> smokers of the world.

You need a little neonatology to get the whole picture (It won't hurt.). Dr. R.L. Naeye, in his textbook on neonatology, reported (underlining courtesy of your editor): "We recently found <u>no significant association</u> between maternal smoking and either stillbirths or neonatal deaths <u>when information about the underlying disorders, obtained from placental examinations, was incorporated into the analysis</u>. Similar analyses found <u>no correlation</u> between maternal smoking and pre-term birth. The most frequent initiating causes of stillbirth, and neonatal death are acute chorio-amnionitis, disorders that produce chronic low blood flow from the uterus to the placenta, and major congenital malformations. <u>There is no credible evidence that cigarette smoking has a role in the genesis of any of these disorders</u>." Naeye's study population is the 56,000 pregnancies of the *Collaborative Perinatal Study*. (R.L. Naeye. Disorders of the placenta, fetus, and neonate, diagnosis and clinical significance. New York: CV Mosby Co., 1992).

So you see what I mean? Are these EPAers liars or loonies – or both? I say BOTH!

Windham and Golub, in their study, said: "The document notes, "…at a minimum, maternal age, prior history of pregnancy loss, and socioeconomic status should be considered as potential confounders." Get it? Side stream smoke is the <u>founder</u> and the other <u>real</u> risk factors are only <u>con</u>founders.

They went on to say: "The relative contribution of these other confounders has not been established, but their distribution by ETS exposure status must vary in order for them to confound the association. It is not clear why this would be so with these particular factors." If you understand this, please explain it to me.

And this is by no means a case of doctors' cerebral catatonia but a <u>deliberate omission</u> of the most important work done on chorio-amnionitis and its relation to miscarriages, still births, and neonatal deaths. Dr. DiFranza, in a widely publicized review, <u>completely ignored</u> the root cause of these perinatal diseases – i.e., the placental disease, chorio-amnionitis ("Amnion Infection Syndrome").

Dr. W.A. Blanc demonstrated the importance of Amniotic Infection Syndrome over <u>40 years ago</u>. (Pathogenesis, morphology, and significance in circumnatal mortality. Clin Obstet Gynecol 1959;2:705) So it would be hard to blame ignorance for these <u>systematic omissions of the scientific facts</u>.

You now know more neonatology than all the California EPA researchers combined. Wasn't it worth it? – Class dismissed.

See Appendix: The California Tobacco Trashers.

Ref: R.L. Naeye. Disorders of the placenta, fetus, and neonate, diagnosis and clinical significance. New York: CV Mosby Co., 1992.

DiFranza, Effect of maternal cigarette smoking on pregnancy complications and Sudden Infant Death Syndrome. J Fam Pract 1995 Apr;40(4):385-394.

F.T. Kraus et al, Monographs in Pathology No., Pathology of Reproductive Failure., eds. Williams and Wilkins 1991. Ch 10, pp 286-307.

W.A. Blanc, Pathogenesis, morphology, and significance in circumnatal mortality., Clin Obstet Gynecol 1959;2:705.

There is NO Association between Smoking and Hypertension During Pregnancy

Let's start with a little clarification. "Hypertension" merely means that the patient has high blood pressure. I have no idea why high blood pressure came to be called hypertension -- maybe some psychiatrist made it up. Then it became known as "<u>essential</u> hypertension." I don't know why the word "essential" came into being either -- doctor posturing, I call it. Why is it <u>essential</u>?

Now on to the point... this "puzzling" large study examined nearly 10,000 pregnant women. The conclusion was:

"Smoking is associated with a **reduced risk** of hypertension during pregnancy. The protective effect appears to continue even after cessation of smoking. Further basic research on this issue is warranted."

Keep in mind that this is not the same as toxemia of pregnancy (eclampsia) that's always associated with hypertension. This is simply "hypertension of pregnancy" without a known cause. But the finding was the same – **NO RELATIONSHIP TO SMOKING**. That's all you have to remember and it will probably be on the final exam (if you ever get to it).

Ref: Am J Obstetrics Gynecology 1999;181.

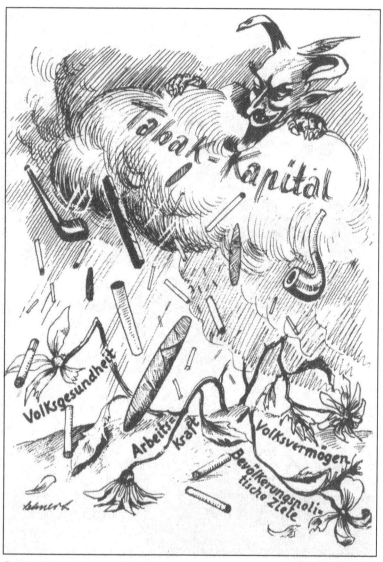

Capitalist tobacco is ruining everything. Hitler was always going after the capitalists. Hitler was actually a communist with a racial plan.

CHAPTER 4
<u>Cancer</u>

Blaming Smoking Instead of Radiation

In the early days of X-Ray therapy, now called radiation therapy, the radiologists were absolutely, positively convinced that X-radiation was completely safe in any reasonable dose. But as the old timers began to die of cancer, the "reasonable dose" kept falling. Young radiologists today know little of the old days and are just as cock-sure today as the now deceased radiologists were then. For that reason, little attention is paid to the findings of Dr. John Gofman, a distinguished full professor from the University of California. Dr. Gofman has no axe to grind; he is retired; he has never worked for Big Tobacco.

Dr. Gofman reports data that should chill the heart of every radiologist, X-ray manufacturer, and <u>every American</u> who is not brain dead. He states that ionizing radiation -- <u>in even low-dose medical applications</u> -- is a <u>necessary</u> co-factor in the majority of cases of both cancer and ischemic heart disease.

The data for 1993 reveals that radiation was a co-factor in 63% of the deaths from <u>ischemic heart disease</u> in males and in 78% of females.

The percentages were equally horrendous for <u>cancer deaths</u>--radiation was a co-factor in 74% of male cancer deaths and 50% of all female cancer deaths.

Dr Gofman thinks smoking is an important co-factor in lung cancer. But, he asserts, it is not as significant a co-factor *as* <u>medical radiation</u>. To have this great scientist ignored by the medical and government establishments, when he presents such momentous findings, is nothing short of <u>criminal negligence</u>.

There are many co-factors that have never been considered by the medical mafia or the government Ministry of Truth and Virtue. Among them are fluoridated and chlorinated water, soy and other vegetarian diets, excessive sugar intake, folate or vitamin D deficiency, aspartame, natural sunlight deprivation, and artificial light. None of these have been considered because it has been decided -- smoking is the <u>Number One</u> pollutant on the earth, bigger than acid rain, the ozone hole and nuclear winter (remember nuclear winter?), worse than industrial pollution and Joe McCarthy. There is one clear and just goal, full of justice, awe, and piety: the elimination of the <u>last smoker</u>, even if we have to KILL him for the public good.

See Appendix: Blaming Smoking and Radiation.

Breast

A study in the *Journal of the National Cancer Institute* (May 20, 1998) reported that carriers of a particular gene mutation (which predisposes the carrier to breast cancer) who smoked cigarettes for more than 4 pack years (i.e., number of packs per day multiplied by the number of years of smoking) were found to have <u>a statistically significant 54 percent decrease in breast cancer</u> incidence when compared with carriers who never smoked. This study is obviously "statistically significant." However, it was a study with only 300 cases and is thus too small to draw any conclusions.

Never the less, this is astounding, especially coming from the Journal of the National Cancer Institute.

Ref: Journal of the National Cancer Institute, 5/20/98.

Cigarettes May Have an Upside_http://www.forces.org/evidence/files/brea.htm

Skin

The bizarre and unexpected findings of the therapeutic advantages of tobacco smoke extend even to rare forms of cancer. Kaposi's sarcoma is a rare, fatal form of skin cancer that affects primarily elderly men of Italian, Greek and Jewish ancestry. These findings were reported by researcher Dr. James Goedertat, from the National Cancer Institute (NCI) publication, of all places – Enemy Number One to all smokers. Goedert quickly reassured his colleagues he had not jumped ship by stating that he was not recommending this cohort of men take up smoking. Well, why not take up smoking if cigars are the delivery system of choice for a terrible and fatal disease? Tell us, James, what course of prevention has the NCI to offer? I think he knows.

Thyroid

As preposterous as it may sound, the reports on the forms of cancer improved or possibly prevented by tobacco smoke continues to expand. Now it has been reported that thyroid cancer, found primarily in women, is significantly less common in women who smoke.

"Both smoking and alcohol consumption may influence thyroid function, although the nature of these relations is not well understood. We examined the influence of tobacco and alcohol use on papillary thyroid cancer in a population-based case-control study."

A history of ever having smoked more than 100 cigarettes was associated with a reduced risk of disease This reduction in risk was most evident in current smokers. Women who reported they had ever consumed 12 or more alcohol-containing drinks within a year were also at reduced risk. Similar to the association noted with smoking, the reduction in risk was primarily present among current alcohol consumers. The associations we observed, if not due to chance, may be related to actions of cigarette smoking and alcohol consumption that reduce thyroid cell proliferation through effects on thyroid stimulating hormone, estrogen, or other mechanisms.

People who smoke usually also imbibe in alcoholic drinks but, contrariwise, many people who drink do not smoke. So this study, although of extreme interest, has two variables that make it impossible to determine which factor is responsible for the protective effect – or is it the combination of alcohol and tobacco that is causative in protecting against thyroid cancer? It is not known how smoking or alcohol consumption affects the function of the thyroid but it is known that they both do indeed have an effect. This study confirms that.

Ref: Risk of papillary thyroid cancer in women in relation to smoking and alcohol consumption. http://www. ncbi. nlm. nih.gov/entrez/query. f c g i ? d b = P u b M e d & c m d = Retrieve&list_uids=10615843&dopt=Abstract

The Cause or not the Cause?
That is the Question

Dr. Hans J. Eysenck, professor of psychology at the Institute of Psychiatry, University of London, has been studying the smoking issue and its relationship to cancer for many years. "A widely accepted theory asserts that cigarette smoking causes lung cancer, coronary heart disease, and many other diseases with which it is statistically linked," he says, but "… such a theory is far from proven."

The current theory – actually a <u>religious belief</u> among its proponents, is that smoking is causal to lung cancer. Smoking causes lung cancer – period. This has not been proven but, it is believed, no proof is necessary because everybody knows it is true and it is obvious. Professor Eysenck gives it the "Scotch Verdict," NOT PROVEN.

"If the causal theory is true," he explains, "then we would expect a definite dose-response relationship; in other words, the heavy smoker should be stricken with cancer earlier than the light smoker. <u>Yet the amount smoked makes no appreciable difference</u> to the mean age at which the person is reported first to the clinic. Again, inhalation should make lung cancer much more likely than smoking without inhaling, yet the files show if, anything, <u>an opposite trend</u>. These two observations are difficult to reconcile with the causal theory of smoking.

"A widely accepted theory asserts that cigarette smoking causes lung cancer, coronary heart disease, and many other diseases with which it is statistically linked. It is not always realized that (a) such a theory is far from proven, and is beset by many anomalies and doubts, and that (b) there is an alternative theory, which is based on undeniable facts, which are not explained by the causal theory. The present position seems to be that either theory may explain the tragic incidence of lung cancer and coronary heart disease …

or that both may be needed to complement each other. <u>There is agreement that smoking is neither a necessary nor a sufficient cause of lung cancer</u>.

"Of 100 heavy smokers, less than 10 will develop lung cancer; hence smoking is not a sufficient cause. And of 100 people who develop lung cancer, approximately 10 will be non-smokers: hence smoking is not a necessary cause. This simple fact (the precise numbers differ of course from country to country) indicates that with routine diagnosis, we find that prior to World War I, out of 100 people found on autopsy to have died of lung cancer, only 3 were so diagnosed. This is typical of the very obvious under-diagnosis of lung cancer then prevalent. In recent years, exactly the opposite has been found, namely an over-diagnosis of lung cancer of up to 200% and more. Whether these changes in diagnostic preference are completely responsible for the alleged tremendous increase in lung cancer over the years or not, and whether it may in part account for the observed correlation between lung cancer and smoking, it is impossible to say; <u>all we can say is that the basic data is completely unreliable and the statistics based on them are suspect</u>." [Underlining added]

Professor Eysenck's credentials are too long to repeat here. Trust me when I say he has 100 percent credibility. It seems that the anti-smokers are unaware that the professor exists, if you can believe it, which I cannot. I recommend Dr. Eysenck's book. It is a voice of calm and reason. My quotes here are only a small part of the book. Apparently, the book is unavailable but, because of the wonders of the Internet, a large part of it has been excerpted at: http://tobaccodocuments. org/lor/03607681-7692.html. I recommend that you read it.

Does Smoking Prevent Cancer?

I heard from Michael Gilson De Lemos ("MG" to his friends) that a distinguished cancer specialist he met in Spain once made the preposterous suggestion to him that some pollution may be good for you. Having an iconoclastic nature, I used to have a bumper sticker on my car, back in the 60s (I have been repulsed by the enviro-coo coos for 40 years) that asserted: "POLUTION – Give it a Chance!" I was just kidding, of course, but I was fed up with all the silly science, posing as the real thing and injuring the environment as a result.

I asked my best friend, in Russia, the inimitable Doctor Nikolai Chaika (Russian for Sea Gull), "Nikolai, how can you survive the pollution here – the water, the air and the God-awful food?" He replied, "Well Beel, we have very strong immune systems; the rest are dead." Sea Gull loved to joke with a straight face. But he had a good point or at least part of a point. It's the old Darwin theory taken to the extreme. Actually the thought didn't originate with Darwin. If Darwin ever had an original thought, it has not been revealed as yet.

Will smoking alleviate or prevent asthma? Obesity? (YES!) Alzheimer's and LUNG CANCER? These questions are so counter intuitive that I expect to get locked up any day now. (I keep my doors locked and my cigars in a box, ready for a rapid, smoke-free exit.) Did the burgeoning anti-smoke horror-story industry have serious technical defects in their research, "MG" asked the professor.

"You have no idea," he replied, "for there's no evidence that smoking causes anything in moderate doses other than researcher's salaries. It may even extend life as part of a complex of healthy behaviors. It may be dangerous but life-style factors, e.g., poor diet, set it off. But no one wants to hear. Moderate smoking may harm, but evidence, statistically, is the reverse."

Here is part of the conclusion that MG makes, based on the professor's cogent remarks and his own experience. The underlining is mine because, well, I like to underline things:

"We're built for stress. Total rest and quiet, cause adverse symptoms. Through history we've lived in high-smoke environments. Smoke-filled huts sheltered us from brush fire haze. The starting point should be we're actually adapted to a level of smoke. Yet there are no comparison studies of a smoke-free environment's potential ill effects. These could be as severe as putting gravity-accustomed humans in gravity-free space, where they soon degenerate. No baseline comparison exists. Theoretically, the stress of increasing smoke-free environments may be a cancer factor. The control population remains unstudied."

I enthusiastically recommend the entire article – see reference below.

****

Michael Gilson De Lemos ("MG") is on the Executive Committee of the US Libertarian Party, and also coordinates the Libertarian International Organization. Retired as a Fortune 100 management consultant, he is working on books on management and libertarian philosophy. His E-mail address is gilsondelemos@msn.com

Ref: The Laissez Faire City Times, Vol 5, No 4, January 22, 2001.

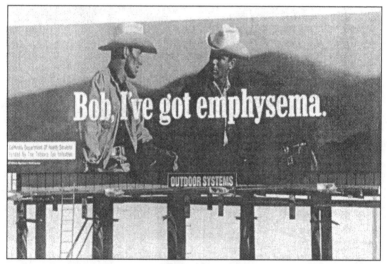

…from cigarettes, of course

CHAPTER 5

Other Diseases and Conditions

Gulf War Syndrome - Blame it on Tobacco!

Sounds like a song we've heard before... everything but the truth! We were told, for example, that there had been 1,124 casualties during Gulf War II. But now we are told more <u>than 6,000</u> service members have been sent back to either Germany or the US "due to medical reasons." (Washington Post, 9/03) That's over <u>five times</u> the formerly reported number of casualties. (Close enough for government work.) These numbers will be much higher by the time you read this book.

Sources say that a hundred of these soldiers have died and it is being called "pneumonia," which doesn't tell you much – and that is the purpose – to tell you as little as possible. Then they say something highly significant; they mention "toxic shock." This means pus in the blood, to put it indelicately, and usually death. Next comes the most preposterous part of the reports I have read. <u>It is implied that the soldiers taking up smoking after entering the army may have caused this horrendous infection!</u> So THAT'S what killed those 60,000 young men in Vietnam. I always suspected it. It wasn't the Viet Cong; it was Phillip Morris.

The soldiers are going "months at a time" with inadequate water in 120-degree weather and "lack access to regular food." This came to me second hand and I don't believe it. It sounds like something the New York Times would come up with. "There is enough depleted uranium expended in Iraq to cause many health problems..." Where does the mainstream media get its science advice – Greenpeace? There is no justification for such an assertion.

But some of the questions they raise are worth considering. Did the massive immunizations they were forced to endure lower their immune resistance so that staphylococcal or strep pneumonia could not be resisted resulting in toxic shock syndrome and death? The American Army doctors in Germany have been ordered to not make comments about toxic shock. Why do you suppose these doctors are being muzzled – for "national security"?

See Appendix: Gulf War Syndrome - Blame it on Tobacco!

Gums

Does Smoking Cause Shrinkage of the Gums?

Since smoking has been blamed for everything from ear infections to insanity, it was only a matter of time before the tobacco phobics went to the mouth for a second look. After all, we absolutely positively know that smoking causes stomach cancer, throat cancer, cavities, cancer of the tongue, and bad breathe but what about the gum shrinkage? Naturally, somebody was able to come up with one of those "strongly associated" studies that weren't worth the recycled paper it was printed on.

Three investigators from Western Europe did a nice study to prove or disprove the supposition that smoking causes "gingival recession," that is, shrinkage of the gums. The aim of their investigation was to assess "the development of gingival recession in young adult smokers and non-smokers." Thirty volunteers smoked at least 20 cigarettes per day, and 31 subjects were non-smokers.

Their conclusion: "Present data <u>did not support the hypothesis that smokers are at an increased risk for the development of gingival recession</u>."

Ref: Journal of Clinical Periodontology February 2002.

Gum Disease Less of a Risk for Smokers

Ask any doctor, dentist or dental hygienist if smoking is bad for the gums and you will get a one hundred percent reply: "Why yes, of course." The study referenced below indicates just the opposite. Moderate smokers actually have less gum recession than nonsmokers. Does this apply to gum disease in general? Any dentist would say no, but with so many scientific reports indicating the salubrious effects of tobacco in a wide range of diseases, we must remain skeptical.

In the strange world that anti-tobacco has wrought, any research that deviates from the tobacco-is-the-root-of-all-evil template is noteworthy. There is no solid proof for any of the diseases attributed to tobacco - just statistics and speculative associations, but the ministries of health continue to lie to the public, in a dazzling display of intellectual, professional, moral and political corruption.

The gum disease scare is one of the "Health Warnings" on cigarette packs in Canada. There is no solid proof that MODERATE smoking causes gum disease or any other disease. These are unreliable statistics and speculation - nothing else. Canada has the fever that has gripped the rest of the world - tobacco smoke is the greatest menace to mankind (and even more to woman kind) than anything since Y2K and the Ozone Hole.

Ref: "Smoking Does Not Increase Risk Of Receding Gums"
http://193.78.190.200/10o/gums.htm

Nicotine for Ulcerative Colitis

"Ulcerative colitis is a condition of nonsmokers in which <u>nicotine is of therapeutic benefit</u>."

Between the sentence above in this report (<u>"Nitric Oxide Mediates a Therapeutic Effect of Nicotine in Ulcerative Colitis"</u>), and the one below, is a lot of scientific stuff you are probably not interested in.

"These findings may explain some of the therapeutic benefit from nicotine <u>(and smoking)</u> in ulcerative colitis and may account for the colonic motor dysfunction in active disease." [Underlining added]

If you would like to read the entire report, then see "Nitric Oxide Mediates a Therapeutic Effect of Nicotine in Ulcerative Colitis" in the Appendix. There is also another good write up from Carol Thompson at FORCES titled "Ulcerative Colitis is Associated with Non Smoking" in the Appendix.

Nicotine Therapy for Memory Loss

You should read the excellent report by Lauran Neergaard on postoperative memory loss, a condition no longer being hidden under the operating sheets, as the condition is now recognized to be present in <u>all major surgeries</u> to a greater or lesser degree.

See Appendix: Nicotine Therapy for Memory Loss.

But in case you'd like a short version here's a thumbnail sketch:

- "Tens of thousands" of open-heart surgery patients lose significant brain function following the surgery. This loss is usually permanent in at least 42 percent of patients.
- The cause is unknown but there are many theories.
- Lidocaine, magnesium and an experimental drug (pexelizumab) are being tested.

You will note, there is no mention in this report of the positive effect of nicotine on brain function when given before surgery, but why would there be as most doctors have no idea of the benefits of nicotine. It would not be practical to give these seriously ill patients cigars to puff on (too late for that) but <u>nicotine can be given intravenously</u>. IV nicotine would probably be incredibly effective. I hope some courageous doctor overcomes his fear of political correctness and tries IV nicotine.

Report from Dr. Sabban

I have included this report from the New York Medical College only to convince you that there is some very deep science going on in regard to nicotine and its relation to stress. Dr. Sabban is not defending smoking; she is a scientist and not a cigar-smoking polemicist (like me). I think her work is highly significant. Just read the underlined sentences, which is the only part I understood...

Nicotine Infusion Modulates Immobilization Stress-Triggered Induction Of Gene Expression Of Rat Catecholamine Biosynthetic Enzymes

Esther Sabban, PhD, New York Medical College, Biochemistry and Molecular Biology, Valhalla, NY

The relationship between nicotine and stress is complex and paradoxical. Although people claim they smoke because it relaxes them, nicotine can trigger some of the effects observed with stress, including the synthesis and release of the catecholamines and their biosynthetic enzymes. We examined the confusing relationship between nicotine and stress. Multiple injections of nicotine bitartarate (5mg/kg) elevated mRNA levels for the catecholamine biosynthetic enzymes, tyrosine hydroxylase (TH), dopamine b-hydroxylase (DBH) and phenylethanolamine N-methyltransferase (PNMT) and of prepro-neuropeptide Y (NPY) in rat adrenal medulla more than did 1 mg/kg. In the locus coeruleus, substantia nigra and ventral tegemtal area both doses equally induced TH mRNA levels. However, nicotine infusion (15 mg/kg/day) did not affect adrenal messenger RNA levels for any of the genes of interest, and did not increase plasma corticosterone levels. However, in rats pre-exposed to nicotinic infusions, the response to a single immobilization (IMO) stress was markedly attenuated with respect to changes in adrenomedullary TH, DBH, and PNMT mRNA levels and in c-fos protein levels. In the CNS, the effect of nicotine on the stress response prevented the induction of TH mRNA by repeated IMO stress in ventral tegmental area (but not in substantia nigra) and of DBH mRNA by single IMO in the locus coeruleus. **The findings may help understand Nesbitt's Paradox and explain some of the complex interactions between stress and exposure to nicotine**.

Esther Sabban, Lidia Serova and Firas Chamas, Department of Biochemistry and Molecular Biology, New York Medical College, Valhalla, New York 10595

* * *

PS – In case you read it, *Nesbitt's Paradox* has to do with... well I don't know, I burrowed through the musty stacks in some of the world's greatest science libraries (figuratively speaking) and I <u>still</u> don't understand it. I guess it means that, although smokers become more relaxed from smoking, the physiological response appears stimulating, rather than calming.

BUT, I did find another paradox of great scientific and social significance: while Irish pubs are increasing around the world at an exponential rate, they are dying out in Dublin. There's an interesting scientific project for you – *Murphy's Paradox, It's Origin and Sociopathic Implications*.

Thin Skinned Twins

Dr. Tim Spector, head of the twin research unit at St. Thomas' Hospital in London, and Britain's state-funded Health Education Authority, are convinced that smoking furthers aging. "It's always been known," Tim says.

Spector and his group studied more than 1,000 sets of twins to identify genes behind a variety of diseases. They found 50 pairs of twins, one a nonsmoker and one a lifelong smoker. On average, the smoking twin had skin 25 percent thinner than the nonsmoker. In a few cases, the difference was 40 percent. Wrinkles occur as the skin thins. Identical twins, who have the same genes, would age at the same rate unless affected by external factors, Spector explained.

But Spector did not mention other possible external factors. Did all of these twin pairs live at the same latitude all of their lives? Did they have identical jobs under identical environmental conditions? Did they all have loving and nurturing spouses? Did they each have identical diets? Did the smokers all smoke an average of 27.6 cigarettes a day? Did they inhale?

It would be silly to imply from this study that thinner skin, or more wrinkled skin means a healthier person. But it doesn't prove the opposite either. This study is seven years old. What has happened to the twins? Are the smokers all dead? Are the non-smokers all dead? Check back with me in 20 years and perhaps we will have some answers. And don't let this study discourage you from moderate smoking.

Nicotine for Tuberculosis

A Shocker beyond (WAY beyond) credulity!!

Saleh Naser, an associate professor of microbiology and molecular biology at the University of Central Florida reported: "Nicotine might be a surprising alternative someday for treating stubborn forms of tuberculosis..." He described in his report how nicotine stopped the growth of tuberculosis in laboratory tests, even when used in small quantities. Then he added the politically correct caveat:

"Most scientists agree that nicotine is the substance that causes people to become addicted to cigarettes and other tobacco products...but no one is suggesting that people with TB take up the potentially deadly habit of smoking."

Well, Saleh, <u>EYE</u> suggest it! In controlled amounts, if the TB is resistant to all drugs, especially the avian variety of tuberculosis, cigar smoke in measured amounts should be administered. There are radical methods that can be used, such as pneumonectomy (removal of the infected lobe of the lung) and pneumothorax (a collapsing of the diseased lung). These were common forms of therapy before the advent of antibiotics. If you had a choice, which would you try first, an excision of all or part of your lung or a little cigar smoke?

Unfortunately, most researchers are wimps and wussies. They are dependant on grant money and university approbation. They kowtow, or risk loss of respect and income. They are slaves of the university plantation system. So, even though it is obvious that it is better to smoke than develop antibiotic-resistant TB, you mustn't say it in public. Scientists tacitly approve of nicotine-based products, such as the nicotine patch, nasal sprays and such, without explaining why such an addictive substance becomes *"un-addictive"* when used in ways in which they approve.

Ref: http://193.78.190.200/10c/nicotine.htm

The Blind Leading the Blind

I thought I had heard everything about Demon Tobacco and how it causes every disease known to man from SIDS, to sarcoid, to scabies, to schistosomiasis. But I was wrong, the propagandistic torture continues. We are now told, by way of a "scientific" study somewhere in Europe, that smoking causes blindness. The anti-smoking crusade has gotten so intense (and vindictive) that I am now convinced non-smoking causes insanity.

When I was an innocent little boy, my stepfather warned me that if I did "that," (what the psychiatrists at the time called self-abuse) it would make me go blind. I replied: "OK then, may I do it until I need glasses?" (That's an old, 1930s joke.) If he were around today, I am sure he would admonish me: "There, you see, smoking will make you blind." To which I would reply: "You know, I think you're right. I've been smoking for 60 years and I am wearing glasses. I'd better quit now."

I am dead serious in paragraph one. I really do think the world has gone wacko on the smoking issue, especially in the USSA. I know you're tired of hearing me talk about it but you've just got to listen to me on this. It has developed into the most important medical/social issue of our time. You think that's an exaggeration? Did you know that families have been broken up because both mom and dad smoked? Neither is seen to be a fit parent because they are (presumably) contaminating their children with side stream smoke. (Better NO parent than a smoking one.) Did you know, that in some areas, you can no longer smoke in your own apartment?

But that's nothing. Now there are areas in California, Texas and other states where you can't even smoke in your own back yard. Where can you smoke in those gulags? Under ground? I don't think so. A miniscule amount of smoke, probably so small as not to be measurable, seeps up through the roots of the trees (killing the trees), into the pipes of houses, and from there to the BEDROOM – aaauugh!!

Where do (seemingly) intelligent people get such weird ideas? They get it from the press, which gets it from the research mavens in the universities, who think statistical studies are real science. Consider the whackos at the New York State Journal of Medicine. They say that one millionth of a gram of tobacco smoke in a cubic yard of air "poses an unacceptable hazard" to health. Keep in mind that a gram is only one three hundred fiftieth of an ounce. This is less than the toxic dose for cyanide, botulinum, anthrax or ricin. The press is not mad; they are only ignorant. It's the doctors who have gone mad.

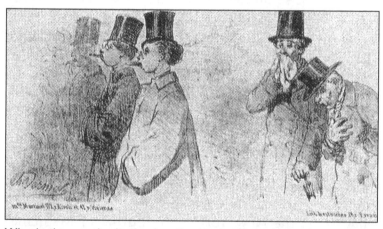

Why is the smoke bothering the bystanders when the smokers are getting a <u>thousand times</u> more smoke?

CHAPTER 6
Apologia for Bad Science

It is clear that <u>excessive</u> smoking is injurious to your health. Anyone who smokes should read the VOL 104 #6, DECEMBER 1998, article in POST-GRADUATE MEDICINE titled: <u>Trends in smoking-related diseases. Why smoking cessation is still the best medicine</u>. We were refused permission to reprint the article in this book. The authors introduce their report with an admission that not all they say is proved (but they believe it with all their hearts anyway). I will quote a paragraph verbatim from the report as it sums up the good and the bad in scientific reporting on tobacco (So sue me) "The statistical associations between cigarette smoking and specific diseases have not been established on the basis of any randomized, controlled experiments but, rather, on epidemiologic data and observational studies. However, the evidence of a causal association is compelling in light of the consistency of the relationship between smoking and specific diseases, the strength of the association as measured by relative risk, and the presence of a dose-response effect (i.e., the risk of disease is directly related to the intensity of exposure to cigarette smoke)."

<u>This is an apologia for bad science</u> -- "causal association." "epidemiological data" (always suspect), "compelling," "observational studies," (even more suspect) and the usual flabby and inept excuses for not

being scientific. But one thing they got right -- "...the risk of disease is directly related to the intensity of exposure to cigarette smoke." They wouldn't go so far as to clarify that assertion by adding: "So, of course, if you smoke in moderation, there is no evidence that smoking is a danger to your health and, in fact, there is ample evidence that smoking in moderation, especially cigars, is protective against many diseases. " Oh no! They wouldn't say THAT!

It is not our intention to encourage tobacco abuse. When I was 30 years old and a flight surgeon in the Navy, I was smoking two packs of cigarettes a day. One day it dawned on me that I didn't feel well and never felt well. I had a chronic cough and was always fatigued. I immediately quit smoking and my health rapidly improved.

I realize that the criticism will be extreme concerning this book as the tobaccophobics simply will not accept anything but the total abolition of tobacco use, that is, zero tolerance. This will have, in my opinion, the same disastrous effect as the prohibition of alcohol in the early 20th Century and the present lethal "war on drugs" which has had the unforeseen consequence of turning our own government into a dangerous, criminal organization.

The evidence in this book makes it clear that moderate smoking - six cigarettes or three cigars (preferably the latter) a day are excellent for your health. If a person has an addictive nature, then they should not smoke at all and they will have to wait for an effective, non-pulmonary, nicotine delivery system, which, I believe, will be on the market in a few years. In the meantime, the nicotine patch is better than nothing.

Return Of The Blob

Oh, brother, now we have to fight Global Drying or Global Browning. Why don't they just call all of these newfound horrors Global Dying, since we are all going to die anyway. Don't go away, read on because this terrible new threat is caused by you-know-what.)

"A leading environmental scientist" – an oxymoron if I ever heard one – has announced that a monster cloud is coming from Asia and will dry up what is left of the Middle East.

"V. Ramanathan, an atmospheric scientist at the Scripps Institution of Oceanography at the University of California, said the major contributors to a world-wide circle of pollution were Los Angeles, Delhi, Bombay, Beijing and Cairo." NOW I get it, a variation of side stream smoke. These cities are killing us all with their side stream belching of industrial smoke. The Environmental Protection Agency will have to take drastic action – calling in the Marines, if necessary – to stop this browning of Amerika. (By Amerika I mean Los Angeles, Delhi, Bombay, Beijing and Cairo – they're all just part of the Greater American Lebensraum, aren't they?) Smokers of the world, take heart, the enviro-coo coos are now going to pay attention to the Great Browning at the outer reaches of the empire. Relax and light up – while you can.

No one pays any attention to the REAL scientists, the climatologists, who are no doubt laughing into their beakers about this threatening Great Shroud of Asia that is going to cause us all to die from desiccation. You want to worry about something? Then worry about having to submit to fluoride intoxication, global fattening (the next group headed for persecution by

doctors, the USSA government and federal scientists --
another oxymoron – and a few neighborhood snoops
who are watching what you eat.) Did you know that
your fatness is dangerous to <u>my</u> health? Haven't you
heard of side stream fat? It is your duty, just as
Goebels and Hitler said, to be healthy. Being a healthy
slave is better than being a sick libertarian – right?

Then again, maybe you smokers are <u>not</u> off the
hook – aren't you contributing to the Brown Cloud
Monster? – hmmm, looks like cigar smoke to me.

My editor says I owe you an apology for this politically incorrect outburst, so I apologize.

PS -- These enviro-fanatics are also after <u>your au-
tomobile</u> – you are killing all those whining puritans
with your side stream exhaust. Once they take your
car, <u>then</u> where will you be? They will have <u>all</u> the cars
(for official business only, of course) and you will be in
<u>the bus</u> and a slave to plebiscitarian autocracy. (I
apologize again.)

Ref: Reuters Health, 2/24/04, Andrew Hammond.

SECTION II

TOBACCO, AGEING
AND LONGEVITY

–A WORLD VIEW!–

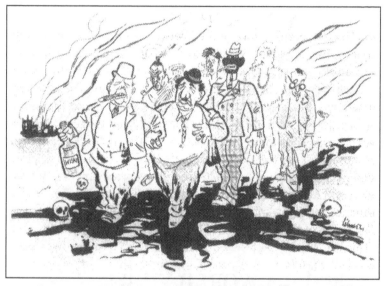

This graphic from Reine Luft equates smoking and drinking with capitalists, Jews, Indians, Africans, degenerate intellectuals, and loose women. They left out Gypsies, Orientals, and Arabs. I guess it was getting too crowded.

Reine Luft 23 (1941)

CHAPTER 7

<u>Potential Gains in Life Expectancy</u>

The world's population is getting older. By the year 2100 more than one quarter of the world's population will be over the age of 60, that's over two and one half billion people! In the developing world, experts predict that the number of elderly people will double in the next 20 years.

But there are dramatic differences in life expectancy in different parts of the world. For example, a baby born in Sierra Leone can only expect to live 42 years. But in Japan, a newborn can expect to live to the ripe old age of 79.

In the United States, the average life expectancy for everyone (whites, blacks, men and women) is 75.5 years. Our Canadian neighbors have a life expectancy of 77. Life expectancy in Greece is also 77. In Switzerland and Sweden, it is 78.

Here are a few other countries and their life expectancies: China: 70 years; Argentina, 71; Ethiopia, 46; Chile, 72; Israel, 76; Somalia, 50; Haiti, 56 and Egypt, 61.

Miserable Gains

From Forces International, we present the following excellent synopsis of the debate over prolonging life at any cost in the light of the simple truth that most taxpayers have no idea what a disaster they are creating with this price-is-no-object approach.

How many times do we hear that, if we could eliminate cancer and cardiovascular disease (all caused by smoking, of course!), we would live so much longer? But have you ever asked yourself how much longer? The average life is about 74 years. If, by magic, cancer totally disappeared tomorrow regardless of its causes, by how much would life increase? Just for fun, we asked this question of several lay-people, and the answers they gave ranged between five and twenty years. In fact, no such spectacular increases would result. If all forms of cancer were to disappear tomorrow - together with an array of other important diseases such as cardiovascular ones (and even traffic accidents) - the average length of life would increase by 15-20 months, and only 15 days for cancer alone. Surprised? Even if everything they say about smoking were true (i.e. that one cancer in three is due to smoking), the increase in average life after the elimination of smoking would be quite tiny. Considering the prosecutorial hysteria of the "prevention" campaigns and their enormous cost in terms of economics and liberty, we believe it is important that the public is given the tools to compare costs and real gains. Antismoking propagandists, who seem so enamored with quantification's based on nothingness, do not seem to worry about educating the public about those realities because that could threaten their power - and that is the difference between information and propaganda. Skip considerations and go to the data

PRELIMINARY CONSIDERATIONS

Some may object that the gains for smokers would be greater than for non-smokers, with the usual argument that smokers lose 5-6 years of life on average. But the loss for smokers is not due just to smoking but to a many other risks that occur more frequently in those who feel the need to smoke - and that often indicate a personality that is quite different from the personality of non-smokers - a personality with an inclination to take risks and either pay the price of those risks, and/or enjoy the benefits. So, if one could control for (that is, keep a mathematical account for) all those risks, the PYLL (potential years of life lost) due specifically to smoking would be much less than 5-6 years - although it is not possible to establish that with any sort of precision due to the co-factors, which absolutely cannot be quantified.

The evident discrepancies between the studies are due to the different computation methods, to different methods and accuracy in collecting statistical data, to different population types, and to different distribution of the risk factors in different populations. What we can deduce is that the longevity gains are tiny even if we hypothesize the total elimination of the bulk of current diseases. Note, for example, that the elimination of Alzheimer's disease it is not calculated. This disease is much more prevalent in non-smokers, it is very expensive from a social point of view, as it renders the patient a vegetable - but it does not reduce life expectancy.

In reality, it is difficult to impossible to eliminate the bulk of the current diseases, and thus extremely difficult to reduce the PYLL - Potential Years of Life Lost. Moreover, the so-called "gains" obtained by the elimination of smoking, drinking, "eating fats," etc. would simply turn into other diseases that are inevitable in old age: dementia, diseases that force the patient into wheelchairs, senile brain deterioration, and so on. That is without taking into account the increased cost of pensions, and other public and private expenditures, often to keep alive those who are basically reduced to a vegetative condition. These costs are incurred in a time where the "right to health" contemplated in several constitutions, a "right" that is as politically correct as it is schizophrenic - inevitably transforms itself into unlimited access to new and extremely expensive technologies and "therapies" turned to extend life sometimes just for a few days or, in other cases for protracted periods - often with immense expenditures that weigh enormously on the community.

The inexorable fact is that the human body inevitably ages, deteriorates, and finally seizes up and dies. Therefore, we may as well enjoy life with its pleasures while we can, without worrying too much about statistical "risks" that are too often not demonstrable. The elimination of those "risks", at best, gives us some extra months in exchange for apprehension, suppression of liberties, and prohibition of our vices of choice, taxation, fear and depression.

We also have to accept that we inevitably die of something. Superficially and rationally, everybody agrees with that reality - but not emotionally, thanks in large measure to the idiotic propaganda pushed by the health "authorities". People are subliminally led to believe that if they behave the way they are told, they don't have to worry about death. But, dying has never been so much feared in cultures as it is today, or so it seems to me.

Finally, we have to accept that probably we have already reached the limit of average life that nature allows, at least on the planet earth at this time. Some make it to 110, but they are rare. We could still gain something by reducing infant mortality, which dramatically excessively affects the calculation of the average life of a population, but that has nothing to do with the reduction of cancer, cardiovascular diseases, diabetes and other degenerative diseases. Unless we find a way to genetically modify the longevity attributes of the population (with all the moral, ethical, social and economic consequences of such fundamental interference with nature), we must recognize that, as a society, we are getting to the maximum limit of the duration of human life. On this issue, those who are interested can read Oshlansky's demographic study "Prospects for Human Longevity", which clarifies how difficult further gains for human longevity are to attain, how they would be at any rate tiny, and how close we actually already are to the limit of average longevity.

We invite those who want to further explore this interesting issue to download the scientific article "Macroeconomics of Disease Prevention in the United States" (PDF, 647K). Written in 1978 by Gio B. Gori (then director of the Division of Cancer Cause and Prevention and director of the program "Smoking and Health of the US National Cancer Institute), and Brian J. Richter, an economist at Enviro Controls, Inc. in Maryland. [Summarized in this book] This article caused much trouble for the authors who, even 25 years ago, made the politically incorrect statement that "prevention" of those diseases that today are so often attributed to lifestyle would incur great social costs. Of course, the authors were accused of cynicism and not listened to by those in whose interest it was to delude people with the paradox of long life combined with "eternal" health.

25 years later, their predictions are coming true. In spite of that, "public health" continues to

deny the obvious, making empty promises and pointing its finger to lifestyles to distract us from the disastrous results of their expensive and futile "prevention" politics and consequent medical meddling.

See Appendix: Potential Gains in Life Expectancy.

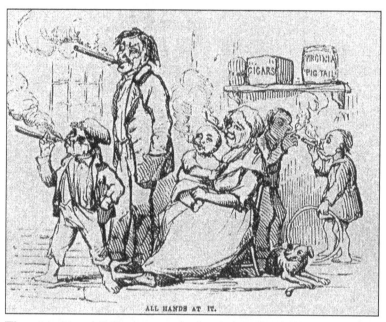

ALL HANDS AT IT.

Those poor children seem to be having a wonderful time. Only the dog is unhappy.

CHAPTER 8

Japanese & Smoking

Here's a comparison between Japanese men and American men that probably didn't make the cut at your local newspaper.

The Japanese are among the world's longest-lived people. Japanese men, who are twice as likely to smoke as American men, not only live longer but also remarkably, <u>have lower rates of lung cancer.</u>

Another way at looking at this shocking finding, which was reported in the Washington Post, is this. The 3.6-year gap in life expectancy between the United States and Japan (76.2 and 79.8 years, respectively) is equal to the gain we would realize if heart attacks completely vanished as a cause of death in the United States.

Now on to the most absurd organization ever formed, The World Health Organization... those un-elected world bureaucrats in the United Nations who are determined to inaugurate a <u>worldwide prohibition</u> against the smoking of tobacco, have awarded Japan their first "Marlboro Man" award. The award goes to that country that most represents the spirit of freedom and resistance to UN tyranny on the issue of smoking. Congratulations, Japan!

If the Japanese weren't so polite, they might ask the question: "Why, with the highest smoking rate of the G-7 nations, do the Japanese live the longest?" In fact, why do the smoking rates of all the G-7 nations reflect <u>the same rate of longevity</u>? Japan smokes the most and is at the top of the heap in longevity while the United States has a <u>lower</u> rate of smoking and its citizens die <u>sooner</u>.

Ref: Washington Post, 8/16/98.

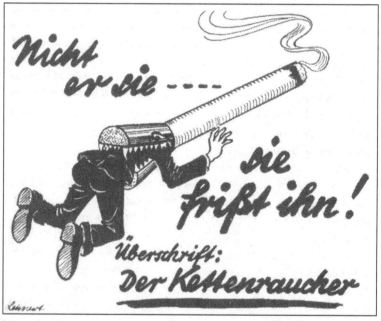

Your body belongs to the Reich, not to the cigarette. "You Don't Smoke it - It Smokes You! Signed, the Chain Smoker." Nazi authorities worried that nicotine created an alien allegiance when your body was supposed to belong to the state and the Führer.

Reine Luft 23 (1941)

CHAPTER 9
Give Um Hell Bell

My great grandmother, Lucy Bell, was the only doctor in Cherokee County, Georgia, after the Civil War. She was an herbalist, taught in the Cherokee Indian tradition of healing. The only other doctor went off in 1864 to fight the Yankee invader and never returned. She was a legend in her time because; as a prepubescent girl, she stood up to the notorious arsonist and henchman (under Abe Lincoln), Bill Sherman, as he was heading south to burn Atlanta. He rode up to the old hotel in Canton to spend the night, dismounted and handed the reigns of his horse to Lucy. She backed up and said: "I'll not hold the horse of a murderer!" Sherman laughed and handed the reigns to a subordinate.

The next morning, he ordered the town burned to the ground, as was his custom, but the hotel was left standing. There must have been a heart somewhere in this drunken pyromaniac.

I'm sure you're wondering why I'm telling you this story… so I'll get on with it.

Lucy was about five feet tall and weighed 90 pounds with her galoshes on. And now the punch line – she was an avid smoker all her life. She dipped snuff, smoked a pipe and enjoyed an occasional self-made cigar. There weren't any cigarettes in those days. She lived to be 99 years old and was never sick. Her friends said that she would have lived to be a hundred if it hadn't been for the snuff.

A woman who even out numbered Lucy in years was Jeanne Calment who lived to be 122 years old, the oldest thoroughly documented case on record. Smoking since she was 16, Jeanne cut down to three cigarettes a day when she got "older," at about 100. She only cut back because she was blind and was embarrassed to constantly ask others to light up for her. At 117, she quit altogether, no doubt because the doctors were telling her she would ruin her health. Barely a year later, she resumed puffing again because, she said, "Not smoking makes me miserable and I'm too old to be made miserable." She also said to her doctor: "Once you've lived as long as I have, only then can you tell me not to smoke."

Ref: USA Today, "Way To Go, Champ," Wanda Hamilton, 10/18/95.

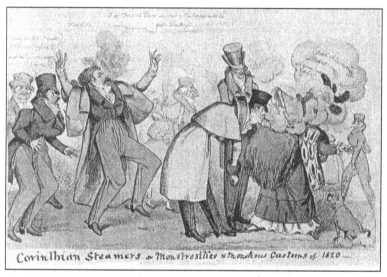

A typical neurotic man who is being attacked by a cloud of cigar smoke.

CHAPTER 10
The 400,000 Who Refused to Die

Lying bureaucrats, from Koop to Kessler to Klinton, terrified the American people by reporting the "Preliminary Report" of the CDC that shocked the world: The SAMMEC (Smoking Attributable Mortality, Morbidity and Economic Costs) report claimed that smoking causes 400,000 preventable deaths a year.

This horrendous news galvanized the American left, right and middle into turning on their fellow Americans who smoked with a viciousness not seen since the War for Southern Independence: "...cigarette smoking is the greatest cause of preventable or premature deaths, causing 400,000 deaths a year, a number greater than auto accidents, homicide, suicide, and various other causes of death combined."

How could you not react to such a self-inflicted holocaust? Fanatics and neo-fanatics came swirling out of the offices, stores, restaurants, and ventilation systems of America. You are killing yourself, you are raising my health care costs, (I could never figure _that_ one out) and, finally (this was later when these pathetic morons gobbled up the Sidestream Smoke hoax), you are killing MY CHILDREN and ME!! It has gotten so insane that it is now illegal to have an ashtray on the premises in an office or restaurant in New York City. Never has the country been seized by such a mass psychosis. It joins the War on Drugs as a serious threat to the basic liberties of the American people.

Is it possible that this colossal claim is a Big Fat Lie? It is not only possible; it's true! You may find this impossible to believe but the 400,000 premature deaths never occurred. In fact, the statistics reveal that they lived LONGER than the rest of us! Doesn't that bring up a tantalizing question? DOES SMOKING PREVENT CANCER, HEART DISEASE AND ALZHEIMER'S DISEASE?

Consider the facts and then ask Koop, Kessler, and Klinton the question: "Why did you lie to us?" Here is what you were not told:

(1) The smoking "victims" lived longer than the rest of us, by about 2 years, 71.9 vs. 70 years.

(2) Over 70,000, or about 17%, died "prematurely" at ages greater than 85. (According to the technical definition used by SAMMEC, any "smoking related" death is considered premature.)

(3) Only 1900, or fewer than 0.5 % of the smoking "victims" died at ages less than 35, while 143, or 8% of the rest of us, died at ages less than 35.

Hmmm, 0.5 percent vs. 8 percent, does smoking prevent death in the relatively young – from murder, automobile and other accidents, infection or boredom? Sure looks like it, that is, if you are statistically ignorant. But that's no more preposterous than the myths spread by the government and your doctor. Consider this whopper: Government medical mouthpieces explained the mysterious deaths from respiratory disease (pneumonia) in American soldiers in Iraq by concluding that they had taken up smoking after entering the military!

Bulletin: Those 400,000 Smoking "Victims" Live Longer than the Rest of Us! Preliminary Report By Rosalind B. Marimont   nce/ sammec/newproof.htm" http://www.forces.org/evidence/ sammec/newproof.htm

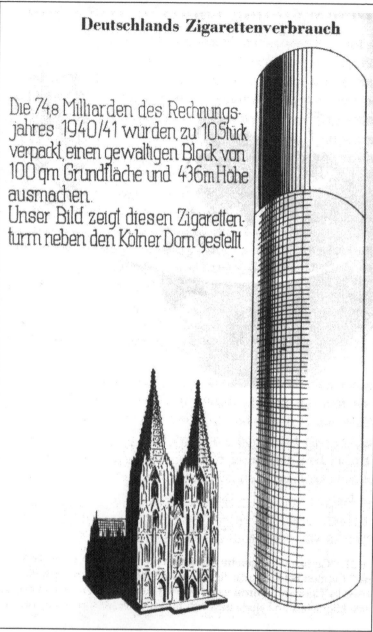

Deutschlands Zigarettenverbrauch

Die 74,8 Milliarden des Rechnungs-
jahres 1940/41 würden, zu 10 Stück
verpackt, einen gewaltigen Block von
100 qm Grundfläche und 436 m Höhe
ausmachen.
Unser Bild zeigt diesen Zigaretten-
turm neben den Kölner Dom gestellt.

In 1940/41, Germans smoked 75 billion cigarettes, or
enough to form a cylindrical column of tobacco 436 meters
high with a base of 100 square meters, dwarfing the
Cathedral of Cologne by comparison.

Reine Luft 24 (1942)

CHAPTER 11
<u>Smoking and Longevity</u>
<u>Comparison Chart</u>

I've attempted to pull together statistics that might further prove the hypothesis; that smoking does not have the adverse affect on health that we have been led to believe, and in fact; that moderate smoking and tobacco use will improve your health. The chart on the following page was compiled from different sources, as there was no single source available that compared smoking and longevity.

The column on the left is a list of countries with the number of cigarettes smoked per person, per year, in parenthesis. These statistics are for smokers aged 15 years and older. This can skew the results, since it is based on cigarette consumption alone, and does not take into account cigar or pipe smoking and is not based on the amount of smokers per capita. You should note that, according to this chart, Japan ranks 4th in cigarettes smoked per person **in the world** and 3rd in the world in longevity.

Country	Longevity	World Longevity Rank
• 1. Poland (3,620)	73.2	56
• 2. Greece (3,590)	78.4	18
• 3. Hungary (3,260)	71.4	69
• 4. Japan (3,240)	80.7	3
• 5. Korean Republic (3,010)	70.7	80
• 6. Switzerland (2,910)	79.6	8
• 7. Iceland (2,860)	79.4	10
• 8. Netherlands (2,820)	78.3	19
• 9. Yugoslavia (2,800)	n/a	n/a
• 10. Australia (2,710)	79.8	5
• 11. United States (2,670)	77.1	29
• 12. Spain ((2,670)	78.8	15
• 13. Canada (2,540)	79.4	9
• 14. New Zealand (2,510)	77.8	22

SECTION III

SIDESTREAM SMOKE

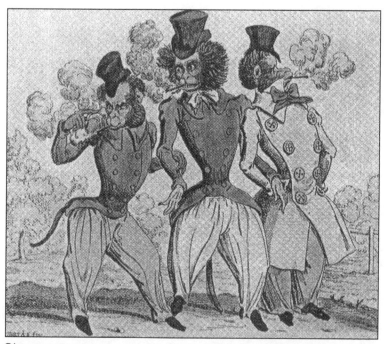

Cigars were very popular in the Nineteenth Century, which infuriated the anti-smokers. They counterattacked with nasty cartoons – only a monkey would smoke.

CHAPTER 12
The AMA & The Press
The Master Manipulators

The headlines screamed and the people went into a piraña attack against smokers – they were giving cancer of the lung to women and children!! The attack was relentless, and the lay press jumped in with sensational headlines:

"What's so passive about passive smoking?"
Secondhand smoke as a cause of atherosclerotic disease.
Editorial, Journal of the American Medical Association 1998
Jan 14;279(2):157-158.

"Study Probes Second-Hand Smoke"
Associated Press. January 13, 1998

"Ex-Smokers May Have Irreversible Damage to Arteries, Wake Forest Study Shows!"
PR Newswire, 1998 Jan 13, 1737.

"AHA Says Study on Secondhand Smoke Supports Heart Disease Connection..."
U.S. Newswire, 1998

"Scary evidence of smoking's danger. Study finds damage to arteries never heals."
By Brigid Schulte, Knight-Ridder Newspapers.
Wisconsin State Journal, Jan 14 1998

No wonder the people were thrown into such a froth with these outrageous assertions backed by amateurish studies that wouldn't pass a 10th grade science course.

A Fraudulent Study

By 1998, the Journal of the American Medical Association (JAMA) had lost all semblance of credulity, veracity, and verisimilitude. Not only that, they were dishonest. Led by Dr. George Howard and a gaggle of PhDs and MDs, the study known as the Atherosclerosis Risk in Communities (ARIC) Study claimed that smoking, even side stream smoke, was making cardiac cripples of all of us. The conclusions, based on interviews, were magnified and dignified by a lead editorial in the JAMA titled: *"What's so passive about passive smoking? Secondhand smoke as a cause of atherosclerotic disease."*

The Associated Press Screamed:

"Cigarette smoking and exposure to secondhand smoke both significantly hasten hardening of the arteries and the damage may be permanent, a new study suggests. An estimated 30,000 to 60,000 annual deaths in the United States can be attributed to secondhand smoking, wrote the authors, led by epidemiologist George Howard at Wake Forest University in Winston-Salem, N.C.,"

But the study is fraudulent, because the authors knowingly left out the risk factors that _really_ cause excess heart disease in smokers and in passive smokers. Howard's boast to the media that *"We threw the kitchen sink at the data, and still couldn't make it go away,"* is sophistic and false. Epidemiologist Howard is incompetent, careless and a fool if he believes his own "kitchen sink" propaganda. Most of the <u>proven</u>

<u>causes</u> of atherosclerosis in the environment and the diet were not even considered in this sophomoric research. The evidence is clear that helicobacter pylori infection, E. Coli infection, Chlymidia pneumoniae, blood iron levels, xanthine oxidase and homocysteine are all, in different patients, involved in heart disease. Why weren't these PROVEN CAUSES OF HEART DISEASE found in George Howard's kitchen sink? I'll tell you why... Howard's sink is unscientific and worth about as much as a real kitchen sink.

See Appendix: Fraudulent Studies.

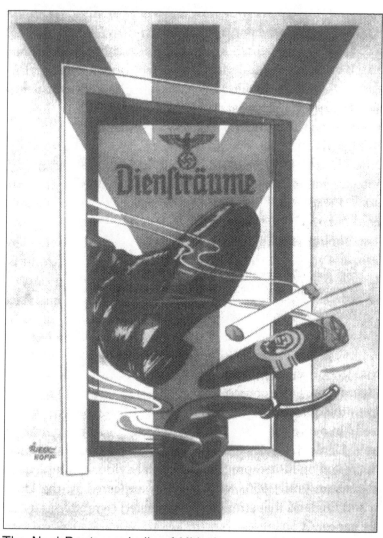

The Nazi Boot, symbolic of Hitler's power, kicks cigarettes, pipes and cigars out the door. Note the picture of an African on the cigar label. Africans are more degenerate than whites and so they smoke more than whites – right? (Wrong).

(Auf der Wacht 58 – 1941)

CHAPTER 13

No Association Between Heart Disease and Sidestream Smoke

The following report titled "Environmental Tobacco Smoke and Coronary Heart Syndromes: Absence of an Association" by Dr. Gio Batta Gori Is the most important document I have read exploding the myth of "side stream smoke" causing lung or heart disease. It is from the highly respected journal, Regulatory Toxicology and Pharmacology 21, 281-295 (1995). My editor threw up her hands, remarking that it was too scientific for anyone to understand. We are reprinting the complete abstract in the appendix for the scientifically inclined and the following is a simplified version. If your friends are skeptical about the premises of this book, just have them read this report. If they are not then convinced of the absurdity of the side stream smoke propaganda, then forget them and blow your health-enhancing smoke in a different direction. If you want to skip the details, go to Dr. Gori's conclusions at the end of this chapter.

In scientific terms, "side stream smoke," passive smoke," and "secondary smoke," is called Environmental Tobacco Smoke or Environmentally Transmitted Smoke. In either case the initials are the same: ETS, and this will be used in this translation of the Gori report. The other important term that Dr. Gori uses is MS for mainstream smoke. It is important to note that this publication, the RTP, is of the utmost reliability in the field of toxicology – they are non-political; toxicology is what they care about. They do not do telephone-survey science. They do not equivocate with "it appears..." "The majority of investigators believe..." Meta-analysis indicates that..." or any other squishy rhetoric that would cloud the science of toxicology. They do not deal in psychiatry, epidemiology, or "public health." They are believable.

This report starts out with a bold and unequivocal criticism of previous literature reviews on the subject of ETS: "Several reviews have attempted to appraise the literature on environmental tobacco smoke (ETS) and coronary heart disease (CHD)... In general these reviews have been selective and conjectural and have failed to account for the many pertinent considerations that a scientific evaluation requires... this present review strives for a comprehensive evaluation of available knowledge by avoiding assumptions and standing by the evidence."

The author gets to basics: "Despite similarities... ETS has composition and physical characteristics different from the mainstream smoke (MS) that active smokers inhale and appears more relatively chemically inert and less biologically active. ETS doses to nonsmokers are small and often below the sensitivity of detection technologies, and these doses are several orders of magnitude less than MS doses in active smokers". (emphasis added)

This means that the amount of smoke inhaled is so small that it is impossible to detect it with the best equipment available and so is of no significance whatsoever. "Orders of magnitude" mean a colossal difference, like comparing a drop of water to the entire water supply of Lake Superior.

ETS and Active Smoking

Dr. Gori further states, "Mainstream smoke -- inhaled directly by smokers -- is concentrated and confined to the moist environment of mouth, throat, and lung. Its higher gas-phase concentrations favor larger respirable particles that condense and retain more water and volatiles. By contrast, ordinary ETS is over 100,000 times more diluted, with much lower humidity and extremely low concentrations of volatiles."

The author points out that, due to rapid evaporation in the air around the smoker, within fractions of seconds from their generation, the particles of smoke attain sizes 50 to 100 times smaller than their mainstream counterparts. Thus the particles quickly disintegrate from oxidation, dehydration, and absorption to surfaces in the room, and amount to nothing by the time they reach a bystander.

Of the several thousand components identified in mainstream smoke, only about 20 ETS components have been identified directly under field conditions due to extreme dilutions. Because of even greater dilution, only in natural settings, most ETS components are below the sensitivity of current analytical capabilities (Guerin et al., 1987; Baker and Proctor.1990).

Compilers of ETS reports from the National Academy of Sciences (NAS, 1986), the U.S. Surgeon General (USSG, 1986), and the Environmental Protection Agency (USEPA, 1992c) have been forced to infer the presence of ETS components "by proxy," which means their opinions are not based on their own research but on the work of other (unscientific) investigators.

Estimating ETS Exposure
–The Hypocrisy of the EPA–

ETS exposure has been compared with current federal standards of permissible occupational exposure to several smoke components. Considering an unventilated room of 3533 cubic feet, the number of cigarettes that would have to be burned before reaching official threshold limit values varies from 1170 cigarettes for methylchlorided, to 13,300 cigarettes for benzene, to 222,000 cigarettes for benzopyrene, to 1,000,000 cigarettes for toluene (Gori and Mantel, 1991). This is in contrast to the preposterous claims of one EPA official who said: "When a person stands next to a smoker he is getting the equivalent smoke toxins of one-half a cigarette." (!) (paraphrased)

To emphasize the absurdity of the claims of the side-stream salesmen, Dr. Gori explicates: " For the average ETS-exposed individual, this estimate translates into an annual dose equivalent of far less than the mainstream smoke of <u>one cigarette evenly dispersed over a 12-month period"</u> (Gori and Mantel, 1991).

Could Minute ETS Exposures Pose a Health Risk?

Because direct measurements of the biologic activities, exposures, and doses of ETS are so problematic, initial attempts have <u>inferred</u> ETS-linked health risks by arithmetic derivation from the APPARENT risk associated with active smoking.

Epidemiologic studies of active smoking give evidence of No-Observable-Adverse-Effect- levels (NOAEL), namely, that at low daily consumption of cigarettes the epidemiologic risks associated with certain diseases become <u>NONSIGNIFICANT</u> (Gori, 1976; Gori and Mantel, 1991). No-effect observations at comparatively high doses are also routinely reported in experimental animal exposure to whole smoke or its fractions.

In a recent evaluation of smoking and health issues, the Congressional Research Service of the Library of Congress stated:

> "The existence of an exposure threshold for disease onset, below which many passive smokers fall, is not implausible." [On the contrary, as you have seen from the above testimony, it is indeed <u>completely implausible</u>. - Ed.] Most organisms have the capacity to cleanse themselves of some level of contaminants. It is for this reason that public policy usually does not insist that every unit of air or water pollution be removed from the environment... In fact, strongly non-linear relationships in which health effects rise with the square of the exposure, and more, have been found with respect to active smoking (see Surgeon General's Report, 1989, p. 44). Were these relationships projected backwards to construct the lower (unknown) portion of the health effect/physical damage function, the observed relationship might lead researchers a priori to expect no empirical relationship. Thus, the issue raised by the potential break in the causative chain is whether researchers should expect to find a significant relationship between passive smoking and health effects." (Gravelle and Zimmermann, 1994, p. 45). [The answer, which they do not give but imply, is a resounding <u>NO, there are no adverse health effects</u> - Ed)].

ETS and Possible CHD Risk Factors In Humans

The title of this section of the Gori report is a bit misleading as it begins with the findings on various conditions not related to cardiovascular disease. But we will follow their format in this summary.

In another of those smoker's paradoxes, studies report that the aborted fetuses from smoking mothers have <u>40% less chromosomal abnormalities</u> than fetuses from nonsmoking mothers (Kline et al., 1993), while other studies report that maternal smoking is associated with <u>a much decreased risk</u> of mongoloid retardation known as "Down syndrome" (Kline et al., 1993; Cuckle et al., 1990).

Studies of human lung cancer tissues found that the various markers for nicotine were <u>not present</u> in 31 of 38 tumor samples. The same lack of correlation was found in white blood cells, sperm cells and cervical tissue. If smoking correlates with cancer of the cervix, the blood and the prostate, why are these markers for nicotine not present in these tissues?

Closer to the subject of heart disease is this report on blood clotting. It has been proposed that increased blood-clotting capacity may "explain" the association of heavy smoking and cardiovascular events. The research, if it explains anything, is that <u>smoking is not related to an increase in blood clotting</u>. The Framingham study reports an absence of cardiovascular risks for smokers of 1-10 cigarettes/day. This included the important markers for clotting abnormalities such as fibrinogen levels (even if they smoked as much as <u>a pack of cigs a day</u> -- Kannel report, 1987). Framingham investigators reported that NO markers for clotting were abnormal for smokers who smoked <u>less than 15 cigarettes a day</u> (Wennalm report, 1991).

A Finish study found a correlation of plasma fibrinogen levels with several psychosocial and socioeconomic variables, <u>but not with smoking</u> (Kubisz et al., 1994).

These are just a few of the many investigations, all with good scientific credentials, that revealed no relationship between blood clotting and moderate smoking. Other researchers have gone even further in exonerating smoking in moderation. These reports will curdle the smoke-free blood of the tobacco haters. There is strong evidence that <u>smoking protects against thromboembolic complications</u> after myocardial infarction and surgery (Handley and Teather (1974) and Barbashet al. (1993, 1994). The ARCS, Arteriosclerosis Risk in Communities Study, of 15,800 men and women in the United States found that <u>smoking was positively associated with levels of Antithrombin III, a major anticoagulant factor</u> (Conlan et al.,1994).

Sidestream Smoke: Cholesterol, Lipidemias, and Hypertension

The Cardiovascular Health Study Collaborative Research Group reports that in a cohort of 5201 men and women over 65 years of age, cigarette smoking was a <u>negative predictor of blood pressure</u> (i.e., smoking tended to cause a <u>lowering</u>, not an <u>increase</u>, in blood pressure), confirming a number of prior reports (Tell et al., 1994).

The massive WHO-MONICA study actually "showed a strong negative association between regular smoking and high cholesterol in the male populations and a strong negative association between regular smoking and high blood pressure in female populations" (MONICA, 1994).

Well known is the so-called "French paradox," whereby the French population shows 55% less coronary heart disease than the rest of the population surveyed in the MONICA project, despite experiencing high levels of cigarette smoking.

The Helsinki Ageing Study reports a slight inverse association of active smoking and aortic valve degeneration in the elderly (Lindroos et al., 1994). In China, coronary mortality is some <u>10 times less frequent</u> than in Germany, although the prevalence of smoking is <u>70% in China versus 37% in Germany</u>. So, in three widely differing countries, different in personality, culture, cuisine, tastes and history, all demonstrate the positive effects of moderate smoking on heart disease.

Dr. Gori summarizes:

"These considerations tell that the active smoking of less than 10 cigarettes/day or ETS exposures are unlikely to adversely influence lipidemic Coronary Heart Disease risk factors. As such, they support the notion of No-Observable-Adverse-Effect-Levels for active smoking and cardiovascular diseases. In fact, the National Cholesterol Education Program only lists smoking over 10 cigarettes/day as a possible CHD risk factor (NCEP, 1988)"

Dr. Gori's Conclusions:

"Plausible ETS doses are thousands of times less than Main Stream doses that appear to have adverse CHD effects in active smokers. Such determination precludes the inference that ETS is a CHD risk, unless we are prepared to forgo all we have learned since Paracelsus about pharmacodynamic and kinetic discontinuities at low doses. By far the majority of experimental reports in man or animals either do not contradict or support this conclusion and together <u>indicate that epidemiologic studies have been chasing an absent CHD effect</u> -- a conclusion sustained by the generally equivocal or null reports from epidemiologic studies of ETS. The instability of data from most epidemiologic studies, the heterogeneity in study design, data collection, and evaluation methods, precludes a meta analysis numerical summation that is scientifically justifiable. The evidence favoring the ETS-CHD association remains conjectural, while the evidence against the association is suitably documented. According to the scientific method, the only justifiable conclusion is that the available data <u>continue to falsify the hypothesis</u> that ETS is a CHD risk factor." [Emphasis added]

See Appendix: Environmental Tobacco Smoke and Coronary Heart Syndromes: Absence of an Association.

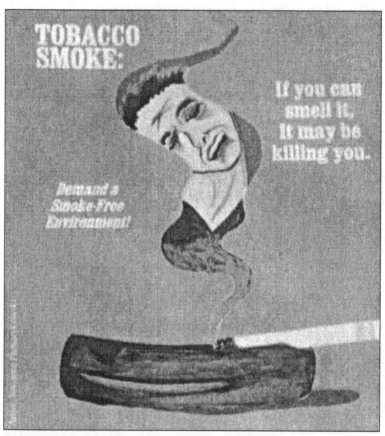

Reaching the height of absurdity – "If You Can Smell It, It May Be Killing You".

CHAPTER 14
<u>New Zealand & Sidestream Smoke</u>

The Blame Game!

The latest world health statistics show that the world's sickest countries are firstly the US then New Zealand. Both these countries have the most draconian anti-smoking agenda, second only to that of the Third Reich.

The healthiest country in the world and the lowest infant death rate is held by Japan, who also oddly enough has the highest smoking rate, of the G7 countries. Italy another country envied for its longevity has a similarly high smoking rate. This revelation was made recently on radio and newspapers and still the zealot's blame the ills of these countries on smoking.

The media doesn't even try to investigate, how it can be, that the US and New Zealand's infant death rate is the <u>highest in the world</u>, yet the smoking rate has dropped -- and why the Japanese have almost eliminated cot death while they smoke like chimneys. Yet, they say, side-stream smoke is related to a high infant death rate. No one challenges their irrationality because every one is afraid of being labeled pro-smoking and, therefore, against the children, pro-cancer, and all the other pejoratives you can think of. Why has the asthma rate in New Zealand <u>tripled</u> but they still continue to lambaste the smoker for this? The smoking rate (they keep telling us) is dropping and, because of the draconian smoke-free laws, asthma sufferers are less exposed to the miscreant smoker. So who are the REAL miscreants? Why are asthma rates three times higher now that smoking is no longer allowed in work areas? Why have lung cancer rates doubled since the beginning of smoking prohibition? Why do non-smokers get lung cancer? Oh, yes, I forgot, side-stream smoke.

It has been known for over ten years that passive smoking does not cause lung cancer. The UN has suppressed this sensational information because this falsehood is the only effective weapon they have to bludgeon smokers into quitting. Like all our bureaucracies, the Environmental Protection Agency (EPA) is completely out of control because the weasels therein understand that the Constitution of the United States has been defacto suspended. Although Judge Osteen struck down the EPA regulations on side-stream smoke as without scientific merit, the EPA uses the regulations to force smokers into the streets.

Ref: The material on New Zealand came from Joy Faulkner, President, FORCES INTERNATIONAL (NZ). She is also the founder of Smokers Of the World Unite. See Appendix: "Let Us have the Real Truth".

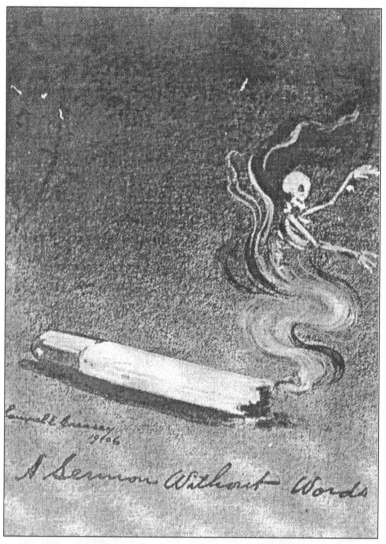

"A Sermon Without Words" implies that the smoke is going to kill the victim in front of it — a smoke-hater cartoonist ahead of his time.

CHAPTER 15
It's All Smoke and Mirrors

One study, <u>funded by the National Cancer Institute, found that nonsmokers have no increased risk of lung cancer as a result of exposure to secondhand smoke during childhood, in the workplace or from living with a pack-a-day smoker for as many as 40 years</u>.

Another study, conducted by the International Agency for Research on Cancer and funded by the World Health Organization, similarly <u>concluded that secondhand smoke poses no significant health risk</u>.

Despite these authoritative studies, and in spite of Federal Judge William Osteen's ruling striking down the conclusion of the EPA's 1993 study, the EPA <u>continues to lie to the public</u> that secondhand smoke is not merely a nuisance, but a proven health hazard.

"The decision (by Osteen) is disturbing," said EPA Administrator Carol Browner, "<u>because it is widely accepted that secondhand smoke poses very real health threats to children and adults.</u>" Carol Browner is a bonehead.

It used to be "widely accepted" that tomatoes were poisonous, manta rays are killers, man could never fly, computers could never weigh less than 1,500 pounds, direct electric current would kill millions of babies, fluoride was an essential nutrient, radon in the home was deadly, X-ray would never be practical, asbestos in buildings was harmful, the ozone hole is going to eat everybody on earth, cell phones interfered with pilot transmission, cell phones will transmit messages at altitudes over 500 feet, a toilet will flush just as well with a gallon less water, nuclear winter will do us all in by the year 2000, the Amazon is shrinking, and according to the late, but unlamented, Eleanor Roosevelt by the year 1950, everything that could be invented had been invented.

Browner, and others like her, applauded Judge Osteen when he ruled that the Food and Drug Administration has the authority to regulate cigarettes. But Browner and other crusaders went so far as to <u>question Judge Osteen's integrity</u>, when he said: "The <u>EPA publicly committed to a conclusion before research had begun."</u> Furthermore, the judge added, the regulatory agency violated federal law in determining that secondhand smoke was a potent carcinogen <u>without any proof.</u>

See Appendix: "Has EPA been promoting one big secondhand smokescreen?" by Joseph Perkins.

The Meta-Analysis Shell Game

In order to make their carefully selected case studies conform to their preordained conclusion, that ETS (Environmentally-Transmitted Smoke) causes lung cancer in the innocent spouses of smokers, the EPA used the old meta-analysis shell game. (Meta-analysis is statistical jargon for pooling a bunch of studies together to strengthen your case.) The method of meta-analysis is legitimate (if ever) only when study results are from methods and study groups that are essentially identical. <u>This is impossible to do</u> because the variables are <u>endless</u> – different investigators with different prejudices (and perhaps different motives), different financial sponsors, different socio-economic groups, different locales and environments of the subjects, different motivations of the subjects themselves, different races with their hundreds of differences, genetically and culturally, different governments with a vast difference in their attitudes and prejudices toward science (If you believe the science coming from Russia, China, and Cuba, then you don't understand the way the world works.), the real health status of the "victims" of side stream smoke, not just what they tell you ... exactly how much did the miscreant smoke, and how exactly did he perpetrate his crime. Was it exhaled, i.e., smoke that had been inhaled or, did he just blow it directly into the face of his victim without inhaling it first? Was the victim in bed with the aggressor or was she generally across the room when the crime was being perpetrated? Was she in the next room – or was she in the house at all? Was the house well ventilated, or air-conditioned? Was the study done in Boston, Bangor, Brisbane or Bangladesh? Did the investigators and the subjects speak the same language or was everything filtered through interpreters? Was the purported victim a priest, politician, penologist, or prostitute? We could go on forever. (Well, approximately forever – my report is not a scientific study but an "ad homonym attack" to illustrate the absurdity of the whole project of ETS-causes-cancer.)

Finally, a new paragraph. If you mix apples and oranges, and throw in a little shredded coconut, you have fruit compote. In a meta-analysis study, you have pseudo-scientific fruit compote, which is better described as fruit compost – and the malaprop is intentional. The whole enterprise is amateurish beyond belief!

Grandpa Must Give it Up!!!

The attack on smokers has been so all-consuming that Florida has actually proposed a law that would forbid smoking in the entire state! You wouldn't even be allowed to smoke in your basement - a neighbor could complain and have you arrested by the Smoke Police. I predicted this years ago in my book, AIDS - The End of Civilization? In 1989 I wrote from that book:

Grandpa was one of the last of the great smokers. He tapped out the ashes from his pipe. "Have to give it up soon", he mused. He loved his pipe but it wasn't worth a jail sentence. The new "smoke-out" law provided harsh penalties for offenders. How ridiculous, he thought, after 98 percent of the population had died of The Virus, the bureaucrats run around looking for smokers...

And at the end of the soliloquy:

"... he could see the Smoke Police in their black car driving slowly toward them. The uniformed woman in the right hand seat seemed to be pointing her smoke detector out the window, toward his house. He took the little girl by the hand and turned to the front door of the decaying house. Pipe tobacco aroma carries a long way. You can't be too careful."

That was written 14 years ago. I was half kidding about the Smoke Police. Now it's a reality.

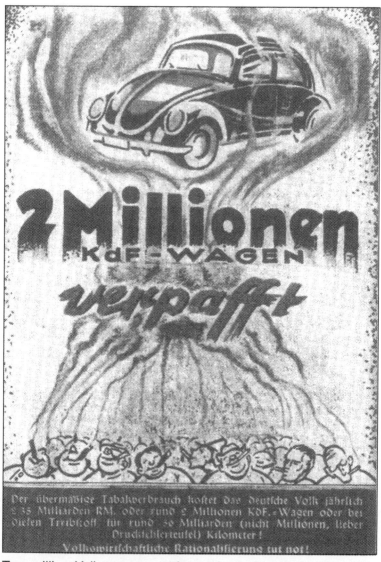

Two million Volkswagens up in smoke every year, supposedly representing the cost of smoking. A lot more than Volkswagens went up in smoke as the German people fell victim to science used as a propaganda weapon to restrict their freedom – just like the United Soviets States of America today.

CHAPTER 16
<u>Side Stream Fat Kills 400,000 Annually</u>

I predicted in my new book, which you haven't read yet, that after <u>all</u> smokers were driven into exile from the Land of the (smoke) Free, persons of fatness would be similarly persecuted and prosecuted. I am astounded that, only six months after I made that preposterous prediction, the campaign is under way. Just as with the national prohibition against tobacco, the leading hucksters in this new crusade come from your tax-eating government. With the tobacco massacre, it was the EPA that led the way with a totally fraudulent study about side stream smoke that threw the masses into a hideous and self-righteous persecution unlike anything since World War I when the enlightened voting class ran around stoning dachshunds. This time it's the CDC, with the help of that government mouthpiece, the Journal of the American Medical Association, leading the way in getting ignorant voters and stiff-necked vegetarians into a lather about people who choose to be fat.

The medical statisticians in the government and academia are long on numbers but short on common sense and, much of the time, they are short on integrity as well. They are cranking up to literally smother us by repetition of the old "400,000 deaths-by-smoking" story.

"Diet and physical inactivity accounted for 400,000 deaths in 2000, or about 16.6% of total deaths.

Tobacco, with 435,000 deaths, was 18.1% of the total, says research in today's Journal of the American Medical Association," reports Nanci Hellmich of *USA TODAY*. <u>This is a gross distortion and a lie</u>! There is <u>no credible research</u> that incriminates smoking, especially side stream smoking, in 400,000 deaths or even 400 deaths.

"This is really a tragedy," says Julie Gerberding, director of the Centers for Disease Control and Prevention and one of the authors of the study. The real tragedy is that medical bureaucrats, like Julie here, are on a mission of mercy to force people to conform to her concept of what people should look like. Procrustes was a mythical dictator in ancient Greece who, like Gerberding, insisted that everyone conform to the perfect standard of shape and size, which, of course, was his shape, and size. He would have subjects brought before him and measured. If they were too tall, then they would be cut down from the feet upward to the proper height. If they were too short, they would be placed on the rack and appropriately adjusted.

"Smoking rates are dropping, but Americans are increasingly overweight." [There is a connection here – more below.] "That's why obesity probably will overtake smoking as the leading preventable cause of death by 2005, says CDC epidemiologist Ali Mokdad, another study author. Almost 65% of Americans weigh too much, increasing their risk of heart disease, diabetes and cancer." (USA Today) And then out comes the magical 400,000 figure but now adjusted <u>upward</u> to 435,000 deaths for smokers in order to make room for the fatties at 400,000 who are rapidly catching up with cigs to prove that tobacco is no longer Public Enemy

Number One – the new serial killer is the serial eater, digging his grave with his own teeth and, according to the animal-hugging, whale-worshiping, menthol-sniffing left-liberals and assorted government researchers, they're going to <u>pull us all to the grave</u> unless we stitch up their mouths, get them on the proper drugs, and send them for re-training.

Do you get a sense of deja vu as I do? Was the corpulently challenged majority (over 65 percent of the population if you believe the statistics) manning the ramparts of liberty when they went after the smokers? What about all those people who are doing too much "unnecessary" driving? And shouldn't they be wearing helmets? And shouldn't your dog be wearing a seat belt? What about those pesky anti-fluoride people? Are we going to let this lunatic fringe deprive our children of fluoride?

"Inactive Americans are eating themselves to death at an alarming rate, their unhealthy habits fast approaching tobacco as the top underlying preventable cause of death, a government study found." Got that? -- "a government study", that tells it all. You are not only going to lose another liberty from this "for-your-own-good" propaganda attack from Washington, D&C, but <u>your health will suffer</u> as well since they will give you BAD NUTRITIONAL ADVICE.

"Poor diet and lack of exercise might end up killing more people than tobacco use and become the leading cause of preventable deaths in the USA by as early as next year, a new study says." By as early as <u>next year</u>? Forget weapons of mass destruction, international terrorism and side stream smoke; we've got to move <u>fast</u> on this one. The only solution is to convince the bourgeois that <u>side stream fat is killing</u>

America. It was remarkably easy with the side stream smoke propaganda blitz because a majority of voters really believe government reports on science. The EPA report was asinine on its face, but people believed it. You cobble up a report, with a lot of meta analyses, innuendoes, "associated withs," and "25 percent more thans," and send this pseudo scientific trash to the p-New England Journal of Medicine (The-Prestigious-New-England-Journal-of-Medicine), or the Journal of the American Medical Association and it is instant holy writ.

OK, so my side stream fat comparison is a little hyperbolic but the result will be the same. Here is the party line as it will develop: fat people are prone to get diabetes, high blood pressure, cardiovascular disease, arthritis, stroke, cancer and every other disease known to man except sudden infant death syndrome. That means they will have high medical costs and, since we now have socialized medicine, we the thin people, will have to pay those additional costs for the fat people. So, as Hitler said, we need to get fit and slim down – look what it did for Germany.

And the brainwashing continues.... THE CHILDREN are being influenced by all this fatness. They see people eating fat and animal flesh, instead of "healthy fruits and vegetables," and they might do the same. There will have to be segregated areas in restaurants to protect the young from meat and fat eaters: "This is a non-fat, healthy fruits and vegetables area – violators will be prosecuted."

Ironically, one of the best ways to lose weight is to take up smoking. And smoking will keep weight off no matter how much you eat. There are limits to this, of course, but I have never seen a slender woman gain weight to any significant degree, <u>unless</u> she quit the weed. Smoking is down and obesity is up. Do you suppose there is a connection?

Dunlap's Disease will almost certainly become a serious misdemeanor. If you get stopped for speeding, <u>suck in that gut</u>, or you may end up in the pokey for a six-month "retraining (read: starvation) program." Dunlap's Disease, for the edification of you not schooled in the medical sciences, is when your belly has done lapped over your belt.

Ref: Nanci Hellmich, USA TODAY, 3/10/04.

SECTION IV

TOBACCO
–THE ECONOMICS–

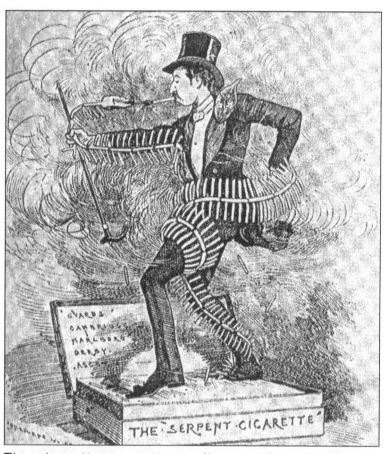

The cigarette serpent – a dire warning of cigarette enslavement. The addiction theme has always been a popular one. If they are truly addictive, how have tens of millions stopped smoking without the help of drugs or psychologists?

CHAPTER 17

The Nazification of American Public Health

Cigarette Advertising - <u>VERBOTEN!</u>
Freedom of Speech - <u>CANCELED!</u>

The muzzling of the tobacco companies in their attempt to promote their products has no precedent in American history with the exception of Lincoln's clamp down on <u>all</u> speech, even that of the Supreme Court, during the War for Southern Independence, 1861-1865.

The anti-tobacco critics became so God-like when it came to advertising tobacco products that they determined they must protect certain "minority groups," from the poison-pen of the tobacco industry. Critic John Banzhaf orated that the tobacco companies, through advertising, "(pick) the most vulnerable segments of society and try to take advantage of their vulnerabilities." The clear implication was that blacks and working females are not capable (due to race or mental defects?) to make an intelligent decision on whether or not to smoke.

Obviously, what you must do under these circumstances is restrict freedom of speech of one of the nation's largest industries "for the good of all." While at the same time, the enemies of tobacco are free to promulgate on TV, radio and in newsprint all the outrageous lies and false science they wish – at taxpayer's expense. As Jacob Sullum states in his landmark book, *For Your Own Good,* the blatant suspension of constitutional rights in the case of the tobacco companies is a good and effective policy "only if we attach little or no value to freedom of speech."

Circuit Judge Skelly Wright said in a dissenting opinion about the ban on cigarette advertising: "The government is emphatically not entitled to monopolize the debate or to suppress the expression of opposing points of view on the electronic media by making such expression a criminal offense." Justice Jean-Jude Chabot of the Quebec Superior Court, who overturned Canada's ban on cigarette advertising, and was upheld by the Canadian Supreme Court in 1995, concluded, "this form of paternalism or totalitarianism is unacceptable in a free and democratic society." Apparently, the powers in Washington do not agree, at least in the case of the cigarette industry. Even worse, American smokers are compelled to pay the price of a government-mandated one-half billion dollars a year anti-smoking campaign. In other words, they are forced to pay for their own humiliation and vilification as an enemy of society and purveyor of dozens of diseases to others.

The blatant propaganda against smoking in the media is often disgusting and in extremely bad taste. Sullum relates the case of a New York subway sign depicting an ugly, degenerate woman with red eyes and yellow fingernails holding a burning cigarette. Above the picture it says: "VIRGINIA SLIME." Below the picture: "YOU'VE COME THE WRONG WAY, BABY!" and blood drips from the hag's picture onto the slogan. As you might expect, this was the work of a high school student. The question comes to mind: Could I get away with this if my subject was Coca Cola, one of the true subverters of our nation's health?

Most of the millions of dollars available to the anti-tobacco forces are through taxes and there is nowhere in the constitution that allows one group (anti-tobacco) to force another group (pro-tobacco) to do its will by the use of public funds. The floodgates are now wide open and who will be next for persecution? Meat-eaters? Nudists? Christians? White male cowboys? (After all, they promoted cigarettes, didn't they? And, by the way, why weren't <u>black</u> cowboys depicted in the cigarette ads? There are plenty of black cowboys in the Wild West movies these days. Don't they smoke Marlboros?) I am not trying to create any problems here. I just want everyone to be persecuted equally. Is that asking too much?

Consider the plight of the smoker of less than modest means, I mean really poor people (by American standards). If you are a smoker, and you make less than $10,000 a year, (A modest income, to say the least.) the tobacco tax consumes 5.1 percent of your income. If you make $50,000 a year, the sin tax consumes only 0.4 percent of your income. The poor person pays <u>thirteen times as much</u> for his cigs. Talk about tax rape and oppressing the poor.

A lot has been made of the "burden" non-smokers pay for the bad habits of smokers. This is accepted by the average gullible American as a proven fact. It was in the newspapers, it was on TV, university scientists have reported it, it must be true and, in fact, it is obvious – isn't it? No, it is NOT true and, in fact, the OPPOSITE is true.

Even Elizabeth Whelan, a rabid anti-tobacco activist, a lover of state power, and president of the benign-appearing and scientific-sounding American Council on Science and Health, admits that it is probably impossible to quantify "the cost to society" of smoking: "...the dollar estimates...are almost impossible to come up with...You can come up with any numbers you want." The assumption here by Elizabeth is not whether smoking puts costs on those who don't smoke but that it is impossible to say how much it costs.

Public health devotees, like Whelan, never report the studies from highly respected journals, such as the *Quarterly Review of Economics and Finance* and the *New England Journal of Medicine*, and *Applied Economics*, which paint an entirely different picture of the economics of smoking. (How often do you read the *Quarterly Review of Economics and Finance*?)

- *Applied Economics*: "Our results suggest that smokers miss no more work than non-smokers because they smoke." (1991)

- *Quarterly Review of Economics and Finance*: "...factors other than smoking accounted for much ... of the difference in absenteeism between smokers and non-smokers." (*Orlando Sentinel*, 12/23/96, pp G1)

- Harvard's *Center for the Study of Smoking Behavior and Policy*: "It is not at all evident that over their lifetimes smokers incur greater medical costs than non-smokers..." (*New Haven Register*, 7/7/97, pp A1)

- *Preventive Medicine*: A 1990 study, reported in this journal, found that lifetime medical expenses are actually lower for smokers than for non-smokers. (*Talk Back Live*, CNN, 3/20/97)

- *New England Journal of Medicine*: "Eventually, smoking cessation would lead to increased health care costs." (*Center for Media Education*, 1997)

The sin taxes paid by smokers are truly Draconian. An updating of a Rand Corporation study by W. Kip Viscusi, and published by the National Bureau of Economic Research in 1994, came to some remarkable conclusions: "At reasonable rates of discount," he reported, "the cost savings that result because of the premature deaths of smokers through their lower pension and Social Security costs will more than compensate for the added costs imposed by smokers... On balance, there is a net savings to society even excluding consideration of the current cigarette taxes paid by smokers." Based on these findings, one could argue, he said, "that cigarette-smoking should be subsidized rather than taxed." [Underlining added.]

Insurance companies are so convinced that smokers are worse than the pox that they now severely penalize the insured not just because he smokes (or even if he doesn't) but also if one of his dependants smokes. Side stream smoke, you know.

And now the smell of Nazism wafts like smoke through the halls of the statist elite. John H. Knowles, president of the Rockefeller Foundation, has intoned: "...the cost of sloth, gluttony, alcoholic overuse, reckless driving, sexual intemperance, and smoking is now a national, not an individual responsibility... I believe that the idea of a 'right' to health should be replaced by the idea of an individual moral obligation to preserve one's own health – a public duty if you will." Hitler said the same thing, and I'll bet that Herr Knowles, like Adolph, has clean fingernails. I imagine that Knowles would prefer a comparison with King

James I of England who said that his subjects were "created and ordained by God to bestow both their persons and goods for the maintenance both of honor and safety of their king and commonwealth. " You might have noticed that he placed "their king" first in importance.

What did we learn from the tragic prohibition of alcohol in the 1920's? –NOTHING! Alcohol prohibition was a national disaster. Crime went up astronomically. Our social and moral fabric was torn asunder. Even Frank Roosevelt, who was foursquare for government monopoly of everything, supported the repeal of the prohibition amendment because the country was facing what we would call today a Columbia-type dictatorship of the smugglers.

You may think I am exaggerating. How could this possibly be as chaotic and evil as the dark days of the 1920s prohibition? Let me give you an example. Cornwall, Ontario, is a little town on the border with New York State. It has become known as "<u>Dodge City East</u>" because of its bloody transformation from a sleepy little town where nothing much happens (The kind of place where you want to raise your children) to a (in modern terms) Baghdad shooting gallery or, if you prefer, "Bogotá North". This is simply a repetition of the Roaring Twenties in, of all places, CANADA! "Shootings erupt almost nightly," reports the New York Times. "In recent weeks cars have been torched with firebombs, shots have been fired into a civic complex on the waterfront and at a building housing the radio station, and the hallway outside a pool hall has been bombed."

The rebellion and violence of normally peaceful Canadian citizens has at least gotten the attention of one Canadian. The Prime Minister, Jean Chretien, cut the tax on cigarettes drastically. "[Cigarette smuggling] is a threat to the very fabric of Canadian society," he said.

But American tobacco phobic, John Banzhaf, who would like to see a tax on cigarettes of <u>four dollars a pack</u>, sees no problem. What can you say to an airhead like this? You can say: "Wake up, John, <u>smell the garbage</u>!" To paraphrase the Canadian Prime Minister, "You are wrecking the very fabric of American society!" It won't do any good. Pinko liberals always promote the very thing they claim to hate the most – Nazi-style regimentation.

Let's take a closer look at the great experiment of alcohol prohibition. Keep in mind that in the old days of the 1920s it was clearly recognized that you couldn't coerce millions of Americans into doing something that they did not want to do, in this case, the cessation of alcohol consumption, without a constitutional amendment. So women's suffrage won the day and, while our boys were dying in Europe to save the world for democracy, the War to End All Wars, America's women voted in the 18th amendment prohibiting the manufacture and sale of alcoholic beverages. Those who survived that ghastly war (500,000 died although you and I were told the casualties were one-tenth of that) came home to find it was illegal to have a drink. Is that what we fought the Great War for, they asked. Is that democracy?

The result was inevitable and predictable. As H.L. Mencken said: "The national government is trying to enforce a law which, in the opinion of otherwise docile citizens, invades their inalienable rights and they, accordingly, refuse to obey it." There was a near breakdown in civilized society. Crime, including murder, became routine. Drunkenness and licentiousness <u>increased</u>. Look at today's Cornwall, Canada, and you will see the future of America unless this new prohibition is stopped.

I predict it will <u>not</u> be stopped because the niceties of the Constitution are now overlooked and we will plunge into a national self-immolation kindled by the Puritanism, which led to the horror of the Lincoln war and the self-righteousness of alcohol prohibition. People do not learn because they are ignorant of their own history. All those who were old enough to witness the devastation of the Volstead Act are 90 years old today. That's not a large action group, even if they were all healthy and really cared anymore.

Let us quote one of the great huffers and puffers of our time, C. E. Koop, to illustrate to you the seriousness of the present anti-tobacco war: "I think the government has a perfect right to influence personal behavior to the best of its ability if it is for the welfare of the individual and the community as a whole." This is Nazi and Bolshevik philosophy, pure and simple.

As Jacob Sullum concluded in his monumental book on tobacco prohibition: "Of all the risk factors for disease and injury, it seems, freedom is the most pernicious. And you thought it was smoking."

Ref: For Your Own Good, Jacob Sullum, Simon & Schuster, 1998. This book is a must-read for anyone interested in limited government, whether you are a smoker or a non-smoker.

These pictures are from a number of different cigar forays around Central America. I was looking for the best of the best. At the same time, I was looking (out of the corner of my eye) for the Fountain of Youth -- I'm still looking. I found the best of the best in cigars right here in the Republic of Panama where I live (some of the time). The manufacturers consider Panama tobacco as absolutely supremo in the world. They don't use it exclusively in even their best cigars because labor costs are much higher in Panama than the rest of Central America -- the price of success. But they do blend it in to their premium cigars to improve the aroma and give them that special thing every cigar smoker is looking for. What is that "special thing?" I don't know because it differs with the man (and a few good women).

I know you would like to know which cigars contain all-Panamanian tobacco but, since I plan to go into the cigar business, I can't tell you. That would be a conflict of interest. I am here to sell books, not smokes. The cigars will come in due time -- keep in touch: www.drtobacco.com.

-- Dr. Tobacco

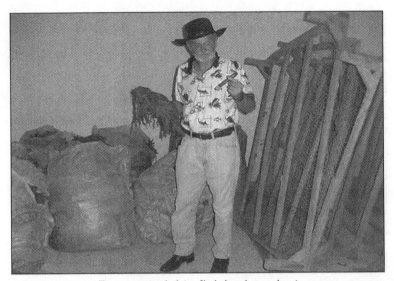
Raw material to finished product

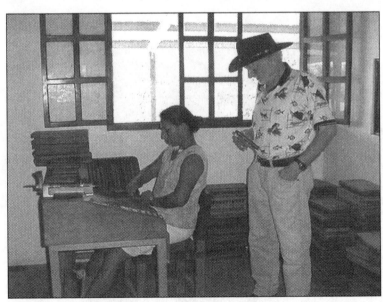
Putting on the "wrapper", (outside leaf) — It must be near perfect to pass.

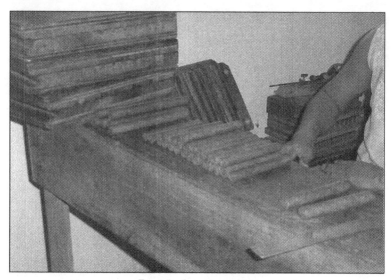

Ready for pressing

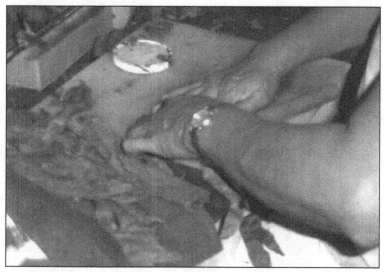

The initial rolling – not as easy as it looks

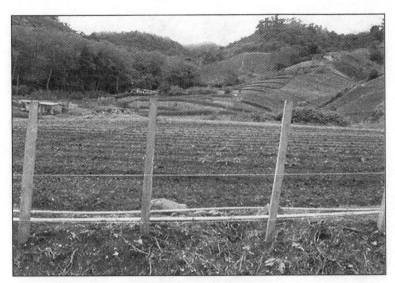

Young tobacco plants

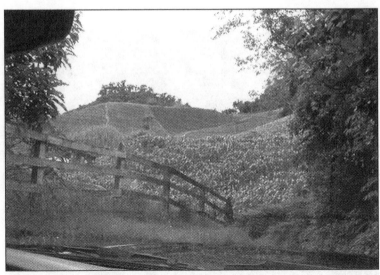

A tobacco (cigar) "finca" in Central America – what a beautiful place!

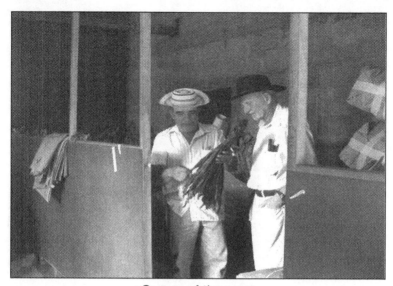

Cream of the crop

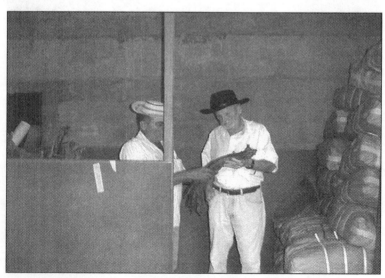

Looking for quality

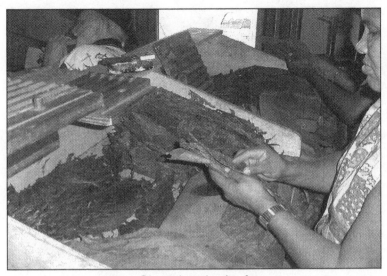

Choosing the leaf

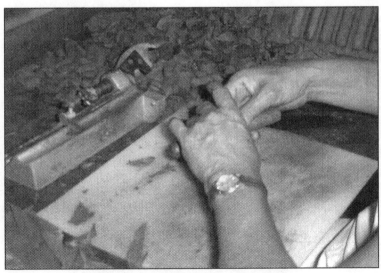

Rolled and waiting for the wrapper

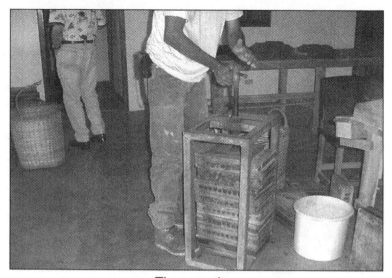

The pressing

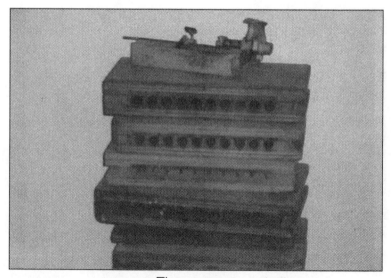

The presses

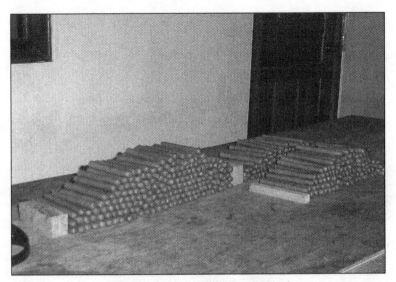

Finished Churchills – yummy!

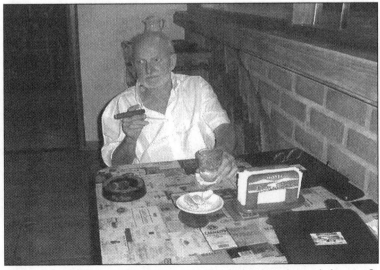

Looking grimly into the future – will this be legal much longer?

CHAPTER 18
<u>In the Developing World</u>

The antismokers who recently convened in Beijing are trying to spread their corrupted science and falsified statistics to other countries for the purpose of launching a world-scale attack against smoking. Among the tactics used is the belittling of tobacco as a valuable crop, and "plans" to "compensate" the growers of the tobacco-producing countries. Of course, their media accomplices cheer the proposal, and withhold information from the public on the devastating damage that this approach would create. The truth is that tobacco is THE most valuable non-food cash crop in the world, and a major contributor to global economy.

We are pleased to join with the International Tobacco Growers' Association, to give voice to a side of this issue that has been repressed by the media. We have also reproduced excerpts from "Tobacco in the Developing World - Second Edition" published by the International Tobacco Growers' Association.

Both their brochure and website (listed on the following page) explain not just the tremendous importance of tobacco as a pivotal revenue for families and countries, but also the absurdity of even conceiving the elimination of this crop. We recommend reading what they've reported in order to better understand the magnitude of the damage the antismoking cartel intends to inflict on the world economy to satisfy its predatory agenda.

More updates and information are available from the Association's Website. If you are interested in the tremendous influence and importance of the tobacco industry on the world economy, you should read these reports:

- The Social and Economic Impact of Tobacco (See Appendix).
- Employment: An Indispensable Benefit of Tobacco Production.
- Tobacco's Contribution to Foreign Exchange.
- Government Revenue from Tobacco.
- The Strong, Stable Market / Tobacco and Food Supply.

You can find these reports at: http://www.forces.org/assorted/tob-dev.htm

Ref: International Tobacco Growers' Association \o "http://www.tobaccoleaf.org/" http://www.tobaccoleaf.org

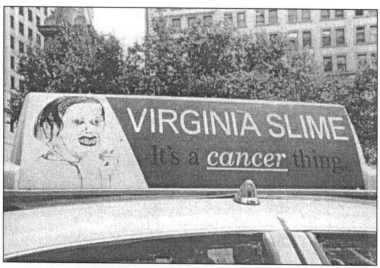

You cannot escape the anti-smoke propaganda in New York and don't dare get caught with an ashtray in a restaurant in that once independent city – you'll get arrested for sending "the wrong message" to THE CHILDREN. Has the world gone crazy?

CHAPTER 19

<u>Insurance Companies All Puffed Up</u>
<u>at Your Expense</u>

As the pressure on smokers continued, insurance companies offered discounts on life insurance premiums to non-smokers. Since everyone agreed (except the cigarette companies) that cigarette smoking shortened your life, this also seemed fair. After the roof caved in on smokers during the 90s, and even being <u>in a room</u> with a smoker was declared a menace to your health, possibly causing cancer of the lung, the insurance companies followed the crowd. Environmental propagandists, often disguised as PhDs and MDs, began to punish smokers by charging them a higher premium because they smoked and by the 2000s, they were even blaming tooth decay on smoking!

Why don't they advertise insurance rates like this:

"Homosexuals and drug users <u>special insurance rates</u>!
Your family <u>can</u> be protected."

You don't see <u>these</u> ads because normal, law-abiding citizen-smokers are discriminated against without valid, scientific reasons. Homosexuals and drug users are not discriminated against even though medically they are a danger to themselves and to others. In summary, a homosexual or a drug user who is free of disease can get insurance without paying a penalty. All he has to do is not tell, or lie if he is asked.

However, insurance companies can now check your blood for nicotine and, if you test positive, you are either denied health insurance completely, or they raise your rate, based on false science! When will the insurance companies start demanding nicotine blood levels at death to prove the client wasn't cheating? If found to have evidence of smoking from the blood test, the company could deny payment, based on the unproven assumption that smoking caused the death of the client – <u>no matter what the cause of death</u>, since smoking now causes practically <u>all</u> disease or "contributes" to it.

Or how about this notice from your insurance company?

"Since fluoride has been proven to cause hardening of the arteries, stroke, cancer and heart disease, we must raise your insurance premium by 20 percent if you were born in, or now live in any of the following cities in the United States:"

The list would include most cities in the U.S. and most towns and villages as well. And here is a fact they either don't know, or won't tell you ... <u>for every person who has been harmed by smoking there are 10,000 who have been harmed by chronic fluoride intoxication</u>.

"We regret your added expense but you can understand the feelings of those who are subsidizing your additional risk due to chronic fluoride intoxication. Please let us know if we can serve you further. Yours, for good health, Purity Insurance Co. (Our motto: "We protect you against everything - including yourself.")

It is a mantra that smokers die younger than non-smokers. "Everyone knows it to be true; the experts have declared it." Yes, they have declared it, but have they <u>proven</u> it? If they are right -- and I am not conceding that -- then by stamping out smoking, health care costs should plummet.

If they are right, then what will be the result? The result will be that these new nonsmokers will live an average of about seven years longer than those who did not take the pledge (according to the anti-smoke fanatics and their statistics). Now reality is that 15 years after the Great Smoke Out, total health care costs will level off at 7 percent <u>higher</u> for men and 4 percent <u>higher</u> for women than they were <u>before</u> the purge.

So if you are concerned about health care costs and don't trust the government to succeed with this "new form" of prohibition, then you should **encourage** smoking. If you don't swallow the government's propaganda on smoking, you enjoy an occasional smoke, and you don't think people who smoke are a threat to the health system... your children, and the human race... then do what you want to do on the issue of smoking. Obviously you are <u>not</u> going to smoke in a friend's house unless he invites you to. You will <u>not</u> smoke in a public place – you have been ostracized from there forever! You will <u>not</u> smoke in a veterinarian's office or a horse stable as animals <u>now</u> have the same rights as humans... except for child custody and theatre tickets.

So no matter what your point of view, you now have a perfectly reasonable objective in smoking – **supporting humanity** and its overall well being by smoking and encouraging smoking so as to get people to die younger and thus lower health costs for the rest of us. Or, how about **supporting humanity** by smoking around people, young and old, so as to improve their health through side stream smoke and encouraging them to take up the habit in order to avoid the myriad of diseases helped by <u>moderate</u> smoking.

SECTION V

CIGARS, PIPES AND ALTERNATIVES

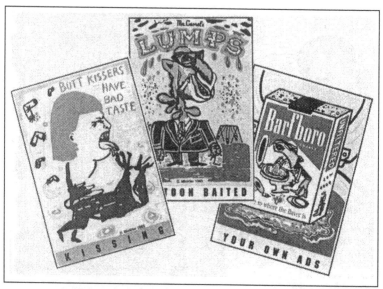

Trading cards produced by Doctors Ought to Care: C. Everett Koop meets Garbage Pail Kids. (DOC). This is about the cartoon mentality of propaganda you would expect from that Great Windbag, C. Everett Kook.

CHAPTER 20
<u>Cigars vs Cigarettes</u>

It's said that commercial cigarettes are grown through careful selection of strains of tobacco in order to have a higher nicotine content than they would have if grown without this careful selection. I understand that commercial tobacco is "sugar-cured" and, if my memory serves me correctly, that "sugar-cured" attribution was used in the old advertising campaigns.

I don't know if they have admitted to supercharging their cigarettes with nicotine but they have admitted to introducing trace amounts of ammonia into the processing of tobacco for finished cigarettes. Ammonia triggers the human brain into receiving a 'kick' from nicotine, which, it is claimed, gives the user a short-lived *rush*.

But in spite of this bad rap on cigarettes, if no more than six are smoked per day, there is no evidence of a harmful effect and plenty of evidence of a benefit. The big question is this: <u>Can the average cigarette smoker restrict himself to six a day?</u> They are a different breed from us "high-class" cigar smokers and, regrettably, most of them can't. But that's <u>their</u> problem and it's no place for government intervention. But the Big Club the government is using is SECOND HAND SMOKE -- "You are killing ME with your smoking." This has been <u>disproved</u> and is so absurd that it is hard to believe that even the science-impaired American people would fall for it.

The production of high quality cigars is an entirely different story. Tobacco used for these cigars is fermented several times prior to being hand rolled into the finished product. The process is as complicated and fine-tuned as the production of a good wine. As with wine, temperature and humidity, weather, seed and soil all play a part. And then comes the hard part, the selection of the leaf, the cutting and the rolling by experienced operators so that your cigar is not too soft (with too rapid and hot a burn) or too hard (like sucking on a ball point pen).

As in the production of wine, fermentation is important. Fermentation is accomplished by placing slightly moistened leaves one on top another in a stack that is usually 3 to 4 feet high. This bale is then covered with a burlap or plastic cover. Temperature is carefully monitored and if the leaves get over 140 degrees, they are remoistened and restacked. This process is repeated two to three times until ammonia and other odors are released. This complex and laborious process dramatically reduces the nicotine content – one of the reasons cigars are not addictive. This also gives the cigar a pleasant bouquet, marvelous taste and a rewarding effect like no other. I feel sorry for men who have not taken up this divine form of the "noxious weed."

Many famous actors of the 30s to the 60s lost their lives from the voracious consumption of cigarettes. Public appearances were very common among famous actors when I was living in Los Angeles in the late 30s. These appearances were usually benefits for good causes. It was a thrill for a teen-age boy to walk around the streets of Westwood village and see the ns of the entertainment world, such as Fred

MacMurray or Bob Hope, buying a pair of socks in a department store – just like us humans!

And so to my point: I don't recall ever seeing one of these celebrities in public who was not smoking a cigarette, even when addressing an audience! They paid a terrible price. John Wayne, Joe DiMaggio, Edward R. Morrow, Humphrey Bogart, Yul Brenner, Nat King Cole, Robert Ryan, James Dean, and countless other "immortals" of the age, died from chronic obstructive pulmonary disease, chronic bronchitis or lung cancer associated with cigarettes. Excessive consumption of cigarettes will make you sick... I have no doubt about that. "Moderation in all things" – what a simplistic statement – but it's true, especially with cigarettes.

And what is the record with cigars? High profile cigar smokers like: Winston Churchill, H.L. Mencken, Milton Berle, Groucho Marx, Sigmund Freud, Mark Twain, and George Burns lived into their late 80's or 90's without getting cancer or any other pulmonary disease.

"The Surgeon General" WHAT a joke!

Your tax dollars are used to keep you misinformed on the subject of cigar smoking. The surgeon general declares on the stickers manufacturers are forced to put on their cigar boxes: "Cigars are not a healthy substitute for cigarettes." That's grossly false, as we have explained.

What does the surgeon general know about tobacco smoke anyway? He is a political appointee. Why is he called a "surgeon" when he usually is not? Why is he called a "general" when he wears an admiral's uniform? It just illustrates the confusion and absurdity of the whole thing. Who needs a federal "family doctor" to scold us about things he probably knows nothing about? He is simply a mouthpiece for the president, the FDA, the HHS, the AMA and the rest of the medical goon squads who want to micromanage your life. When I become surgeon general, the first thing I am going to do is abolish my position – and I will NOT wear that uniform, which is an insult to the Navy.

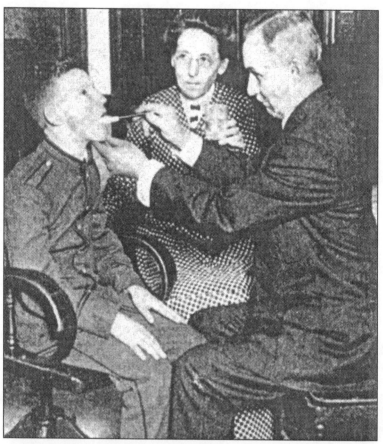

Silver nitrate swabbing of the throat to deter smoking. One of the medical professions more stupid ideas which ranks down there with blood letting, mercury therapy, and moxibustion.

CHAPTER 21
<u>My Case for Cigars</u>

You can read the following report if you like. Or you can skip down to the last sentence (I have even underlined it for you) and get the only message here that counts. (Trust me, I'm a cigar-smoking doctor.)

Cigar smoking linked to increased Health Risks in Men.

Iribarren and colleagues examined the risk of coronary artery disease, chronic lung disease, stroke and cancer in a cohort of men who smoked cigars regularly. Study participants were men between 30 and 85 years of age. These men had no history of smoking cigarettes and were not currently pipe smokers. A self-administered questionnaire was used to gather information on drinking and smoking habits. The degree of smoking was quantified to fewer than five, five to 10, or more than 10 cigars per day.

They reported that rates for chronic obstructive pulmonary disease (COPD) and all cardiovascular outcomes were "significantly higher" for the cigar smokers. There was no difference in the number of strokes and the rate of peripheral vascular disease between smokers and nonsmokers. Cigar smokers had a significantly higher incidence of oropharyngeal cancers and lung cancer. Other cancers studied -- bladder, colorectal, kidney and pancreatic – showed no significant increase in cigar smokers.

It is hard to believe that "all cardiovascular out-comes," were significantly higher in cigar smokers when, as they report, there was no difference in the number of strokes and the rate of peripheral vascular disease between smokers and nonsmokers. This im-plies that the arteries of the heart are affected by cigar smoke and the arteries of the rest of the body are not affected at all. This survey, which is basically what it was, presents NONE of the scientific evidence from peer-reviewed journals, which show great benefit in many diseases from moderate smoking. In this book, we have presented both sides of the issue – and to-bacco wins.

I have over the years, had hundreds of cigar smokers in my practice and I have always been im-pressed at how little of these horrendous diseases I have seen in this cohort of patients even <u>if they were relatively heavy smokers</u> but had never been heavy cigarette smokers. I no longer consider the New Eng-land Journal of Medicine to be a reliable scientific pub-lication. They lost much of their credibility when they started accepting advertising in their pages. They have been slipping ever since they made that fateful deci-sion. As for David Satcher and his Federal health bu-reaucracy, they are 100 percent dedicated to the total eradication of smoking, no matter how much they have to restrict the rights of millions of smoking Americans. They have been caught in so much fraud on this issue that they have no credibility whatsoever. The NEJM loses even more credibility by publishing ANYTHING promulgated by this government propa-ganda machine.

"The authors concluded that cigar smoking, especially more than five per day, produces a moderate increase in the risk of coronary artery disease, COPD and cancers of the lung and upper aerodigestive tract."

"This is a concern in light of the growing popularity of cigar smoking in recent years," the authors opine, but it must be pointed out that none of this applies to cigar, pipe or even cigarette smoking when done in MODERATION, that is five or less cigars or cigarettes per day.

Ref: Iribarren C, et al. Effect of cigar smoking on the risk of cardiovascular disease, chronic obstructive pulmonary disease, and cancer in men. N Engl J Med June 10, 1999; 340:1773-80, and Satcher D. Cigars and public health. N Engl J Med 1999;340:1829-31.

Smoking Around the World

In today's anti-cigar climate, if you have an active and mobile life, it is hard to imagine how you could find ten places that would allow you to smoke a cigar. I was in a little backwater Caribbean port recently with few paved streets, a lot of poverty and a surprisingly good five-star hotel. (This is not unusual in these "developing" countries.) There was a lovely lawn garden in the back bordering the sea with chirping birds, tropical flowers and a typical on-shore breeze. It was gloriously open and the air was sweet – nature's air conditioning at its best! And then there was the wooden sign pounded into the lawn: "No Smoking!" I guess the birds complained!

I was in a hotel at Cape Canaveral, Florida and went to the downstairs bar for a little libation and cigar before dinner. The cigarette smoke was so thick you could hardly see the "No Smoking!" sign across the room. I was asked to leave - no cigars or pipes allowed - and there wasn't a woman in the place! In

Panama City, Republic of Panama, a big, burly, six-foot-two guy of about 65, stormed out of the restaurant bar when I lit up a Churchill to accompany my glass of sherry. The world has become a very prissy place.

A Note on the Cigar Baron

This document is an accumulation of scientific reports and papers regarding the health affects of cigar smoking. It was compiled by Marc J. Schneiderman, M.D., a.k.a. CigarBaron@aol.com. I consider this to be the definitive word on the subject, a result of some very detailed research, hence the title Cigar/Health FAQ. Although I was tempted to include this wonderful collection of medical reports in this book, it stands too well as a separate FAQ. I urge all serious cigar smokers to read through it, and draw their own conclusions on the health affects of one of our chosen hobbies.

See Appendix: From the Cigar Baron.

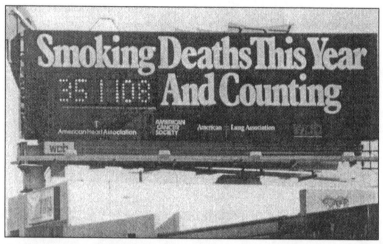

An American Cancer Society billboard in Los Angeles tallies deaths attributed to smoking. Somebody must be really busy counting all those corpses. Don't people die of anything else, such as fluoride poisoning, sugar poisoning (diabetes) or old age?

CHAPTER 22

<u>But I Never Inhaled!</u>

If you enjoy smoking a cigar, and are willing to endure the slings and arrows of most women, this is a pleasant way to get your daily nicotine dose. You do not, and should not, inhale. No respectable cigar or pipe smoker inhales. The aroma is the thing. Women call it odor; we call it aroma. And speaking of women, if they could just loosen up a bit and learn to enjoy the aroma of a good cigar, they could get the same health benefits as their partner through side stream smoke. Or you can enjoy it as <u>direct</u> stream smoke. Have your mate gently blow the smoke your way as you sit about a yard down wind from him. Inhale deeply or shallowly, depending on your experience, mood or dedication to good health. (Think Alzheimer's and Parkinson's, Madam, and you might be willing to give it a try. It's possible you could learn to enjoy a short one after dinner with a little shooter of Compare or Grand Marnier. Ahhh, the pleasure you are missing – and there's also the camaraderie with your loved one.)

Please be assured that the above side-stream/direct-stream advice <u>is not a sellout to inhaling tobacco smoke</u>, neither cigarette nor cigar, directly from the burning leaf. The ambient air immediately cools the smoke, even if you are not in an air-conditioned room. In fact, a smoke-filled poolroom, with or without air conditioning, is an excellent way to get your daily dose of nicotine. Fifteen minutes should be enough unless, of course, you want to play pool.

<u>With the water pipe, you inhale the smoke directly. It's quite mild – you'll be surprised.</u> Let me add, I am not recommending this as a substitute for abstinence for those of you who are addicted to cigarette smoking. If you have quit cigarettes, you <u>should not</u> take up cigar smoking for at least two years and, even that, may be risky for you.

This varies with the individual. I quit smoking cigarettes 40 years ago and almost immediately took up the smoking of cigars. I smoked three a day. Forty years later, I am <u>still</u> smoking three a day and I find cigarette smoke to be extremely irritating to my eyes and nasopharynx.

A bartender may spend half his life in a smoky poolroom. They always look healthy to me. I have never done a study to determine their longevity but I'll bet they meet or exceed the national average. Amazingly, boozers also seem to do remarkably well <u>unless</u> they smoke cigarettes. (A colleague of mine had a sign over his bar depicting an old, grinning reprobate who proclaimed: "There are more old drunks than old doctors.")

I am not recommending that you become a boozer. But science has proven that a little alcohol, especially, but not exclusively red wine, is good for your longevity curve. You want that curve to go East, not Southeast, and a little of the sinful potions mentioned here can help. It's all in the dose and, with smoking, the mode of administration.

As with all foods, drugs and herbs (and even radiation), **the dosage is the thing.** Iodine, for example in small doses is often excellent therapy. In large doses, it can kill you. The same thing is true for potassium, digitalis, magnesium, radioactivity (Small doses of the right radiation are healthy, it's called radiation hormesis), salt, water, and even oxygen under certain circumstances can be harmful or deadly.

It is important to note that even critical, scientific articles about the health effects of cigars (*New England Journal of Medicine*, June 10, 1999; 340:1773-80, and "Cigars and Public Health", *New England Journal of Medicine*, 1999; 340 1829-31), admit that <u>less than five cigars a day are not harmful</u>. I question that even <u>ten a day</u> would be harmful. I have had only one cigar-smoking patient who died young. He was 60 but he had horrible eating habits and was 100 pounds over weight. Many famous men – Churchill, H.L. Mencken, and George Burns – smoked ten to twenty stogies a day and they all lived into the 80s or beyond.

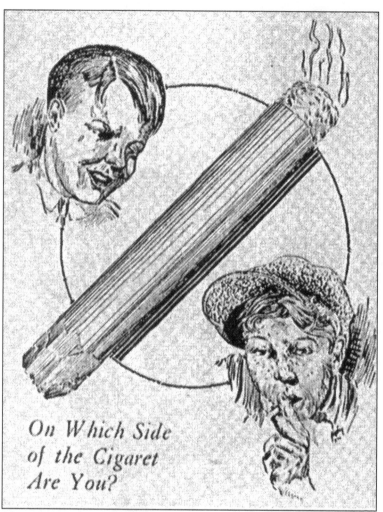

On Which Side of the Cigaret Are You?

If you smoke, your beauty will quickly fade away. Looks like smoking also causes pimples – and dirty hair. "Scientific studies" proclaim that smoking causes blindness and cavities, so why not pimples?

CHAPTER 23
<u>The Alternatives</u>

New Twist on Cigarettes... and It's NO "Ecstasy"!

Everyone is after you to quit smoking. You're blamed for giving other people lung cancer by just being in the <u>same room</u> with them! Now they say you're giving people— especially children—asthma, birth defects, and even <u>tooth decay</u>!

So what's a nicotine addict like you to do? QUIT? Well, let's not panic yet. You addictive degenerates have <u>rights</u> just like normal people. It's just that some people (the new Puritans) think they have more rights than others.

What can you do to protect <u>your</u> right to smoke if you want to? Well you could try the new Ecstasy cigarettes. I know what you're probably thinking, but in this case, Ecstasy is just the brand name, and it doesn't have anything to do with the drug you've heard about on Dateline and 20/20.

It's a clever idea, marketwise: tobacco is bad; herbs are good, so smoke herbs. With that in mind, Ecstasy "cigarettes" were created out of a combination of lettuce, damiana, catnip, peppermint, and passionflower. The burning concoction smells like marijuana but has no mood effects, no hallucinogenic effects and is not addictive.

They are promoted as "100% legal weed smokes" and a way to "enhance your love life." It didn't work for me and I doubt it would work for you. But, to be candid, I didn't give it a fair trial—one puff was all I could tolerate.

They <u>are</u> 100 percent legal, but who knows what inhaling passionflower will do to your mind? And what about inhaling catnip? Before lighting up, send your cat over to the neighbor. Is damiana meant to be inhaled? Do you know what damiana IS? I think you're old enough to know—<u>it's a female-specific aphrodisiac</u>. So unless you are prepared for the consequences, before you light up you'd better go ahead and send your wife off to the neighbors along with the cat.

They're available from numerous on-line sources (go to google.com and type in "Ecstasy cigarettes" for a complete list. Please note that I have no information on or affiliation with any of these sources). In my opinion, this stuff is <u>krapola</u>. But if you want to try it, go right ahead. Just don't let your cat get any "second hand" smoke. As for your wife, that's a personal decision.

Ref: "Ecstacy cigarettes, regular," Ecstacy, Inc. (product description, www.ecstacyinc.com" www.ecstacyinc.com), accessed 9/30/03.

Tobacco Cuisine

For years I have agonized over the nutritional benefits of tobacco. It's a plant – right? It's green – right? I always wondered why you couldn't eat to-bacco leaves - lettuce, spinach, kale, they're all leaves so why not tobacco? Why can't you prepare it as a soup, as in potato soup and cabbage soup? Why not cook it up like collard greens? Does it taste terrible? Will it kill you, like raw tomatoes used to kill in the 19th Century? Can it be used as a salad? I have never had the nerve to try it.

But since the iron curtain has fallen over New York, <u>where it is a crime to even own an ashtray in a restaurant</u> (honest!), the rebellious spirit of the average New Yorker has exploded into a counter attack and now New York leads the way in tobacco cuisine. The restaurants have cooked up a way to smoke out the bureaucrats. At the Serafina Sandro restaurant in New York City, you can order filet mignon in a tobacco-wine sauce, gnocchi made with tobacco, and for desert, you can order tobacco panna cotta. With your after-dinner cigar (Woops, sorry, illegal.), you can enjoy a glass of tobacco-infused grappa. This is all a natural reaction to the Draconian restrictions now in force in the Big Apple (and, by the time you read this, the rest of the state). Yet, New York has become such a Puritanical <u>nut</u> <u>house</u> over smoking that many leading chefs are even afraid to use tobacco flavoring! Alex Garcia, the chef of Patria restaurant in New York, was tempted to serve a coffee-and-tobacco-infused chocolate truffle. "I do Latin American cuisine," he said, "and since tobacco is the epitome of the Cubans, I really wanted to do a dessert called coffee and cigarettes," but "I just don't feel comfortable with using regular tobacco or chopped up cigars." OK, Alex, so you're a weenie.

Smoke-easies cannot be far away. Oh, the fun of it; I can hardly wait. The little hole in the door shows a glimmer of light. A rough voice, reminiscent of Marlon Brando in The Godfather, asks: "What cha want?" The password for today is "cloudy skies." I croak it out, overcome with excitement. "What's ya number?" I went blank. Melissa (a mean cigar smoker for a chick) whispered in my ear: "008." -- "Zero-Zero-Eight," I blurted.

The door creaked open, just as they do in the movies. And there it was! The smoke was so thick you could hardly see the "NO SMOKING" sign across the room (with Mayor Bloomberg's name at the bottom). A top-heavy waitress with very long legs appeared. "Evening, guys, What'll ya have to drink?" Melissa's eyebrows arched up: "Oh, you serve drinks too – how cool! I'll have a robusto with a maduro wrapper, preferably Panamanian or Nicaraguan – and a glass of water."

In the British edition of a cookbook, "The Art of the Tart" (Random House, 2000), the author, Tamasin Day - Lewis included a recipe for fig tart with tobacco syrup. Her editor in New York took the tobacco syrup out of the recipe in the American edition.

"It's an absolutely wonderful dish," Ms. Day-Lewis said to reporter, Melissa Clark. "The gingery innards of figs are not unlike tobacco, and the combination is magical. You have the dryness of the tobacco alongside the bosky figs. It's really sad that it's not in the American version." Her American editor, Pamela Cannon, said, "I just didn't want anyone to open the book onto that recipe and be turned off" -- another New York weenie.

And speaking of weenies and woosies, let's not leave out the public health Big Brains who are about to have an epileptic fit over chefs using tobacco as a flavoring. Reporter Melissa Clark, when broaching the subject to these protectors of our health, was met with "explosive rejection" of the idea of using tobacco in food, not that they could actually cite any evidence of a possible harmful effect. Who needs evidence? "Everybody knows..."

By the way, Melissa is working on a tobacco cookbook. Look for an announcement of the publication in the health section of the New York Times. It will be easy to find because next to the news item there's bound to be an advisory with black background: "The Surgeon General has determined that eating tobacco is a danger to your health."

Ref: http://iol.co.za/index.php?click_id=29&set_id=1&art_id=
       qw1071317701635B223"

       http://iol.co.za/index.php?click_id=29&set_id=1&art_id=
       qw1071317701635B223

Ref: New York Times,1/31/01, Melissa Clark.

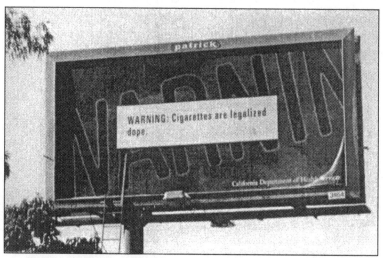

A 1990 California Department of Health Services billboard explicitly ties tobacco to illegal drugs. Your tax dollars at work. Do you suppose they would accept an ad from your author that states: "Smoking is Good for U! — in Moderation." There is no freedom of speech in California (or any of America's airline terminals) and the ad would be forbidden.

CHAPTER 24
<u>Words of Wisdom</u>

There is a lot of good advice in this dissertation, things I didn't know, and you, my faithful reader, probably didn't know either.

Yes there are conspiracies - many of them

"Smoking tobacco causes lung cancer". Right? Well, not necessarily. Media and government sponsored programs pound us with the idea that nicotine is addictive, dangerous, carcinogenic, and outright evil. Everyone is urged to stop smoking, taxes on tobacco are continually increased, and ever-constrictive laws are passed against smokers. Have you ever wondered why the 'establishment' is anti-tobacco? Do you think the 'establishment' is concerned for our health? In truth, there are multiple sinister agendas behind the supposed "War on Tobacco," which like the "War on Drugs" is a complete hoax! Both commercial tobacco companies and upper government groups who are supposed to be anti-tobacco are guilty of collusion, of conspiring toward a common aim which is to exploit and suppress smokers and non-smokers alike. Then there are the misguided minions who take part in anti-smoking organizations to "spread the message" that it's never too late to quit. Anti-smokers can be as rabid as anti-Semites, and it's all by design."

<u>The anti-smokers and the Nazi's</u>

"Now, let's look at anti-smoking organizations. Their message is simple: smoking is dangerous, it causes lung cancer, it contains chemicals X, Y, and Z, it is dirty, it's uncool, etc. The Nazis were rabidly anti-tobacco, calling it "masturbation of the lungs" and a disgrace to the master race. As is known, the Nazis were another product of the 'establishment' and what we see now in America follows a similar trend for that reason." (**See the anti-smoking cartoons herein and you will see the striking similarity between the Nazi campaign and the present campaign by the neo-Nazi environmental movement.**

"What is interesting is that anti-tobacco organizations are just like liberal environmental groups: opposing something without seeing the real solution. For example, Green Peace is against the production or use of petroleum, and yet it does nothing to research or endorse free energy technologies. Likewise, anti-tobacco organizations regularly list the carcinogenic chemicals found in cigarette smoke and yet do not investigate why those chemicals are there to begin with or if there is a better alternative. Supporters of such organizations are naive because they don't understand the facts. They are also heavily programmed by media, school, and church propaganda, and therefore do little more than frown down upon smokers or bark at them. It's ironic that alcohol does not receive the same attention, considering it is far more dangerous than nicotine. Of course, the explanation is clear: alcohol dumbs down the population, something both alcohol companies and the establishment want, while nicotine does the opposite and therefore receives suppression."

Commercial Tobacco vs Pure Tobacco

"The 'establishment' is trying its best to keep people from choosing to smoke pure tobacco. As discussed, this is done two ways: stop people from smoking at all, and corrupt any tobacco products that they do smoke. Why? Because compared to commercial tobacco, <u>pure tobacco has far less side effects commonly associated with "regular" tobacco</u>. Of course, there are no studies that prove this - to do such a study would be politically incorrect and would receive no funding unless the data is cooked to support the Agenda.

"So what does pure tobacco do? As stated...and confirmed by myself and anyone else who has tried it, natural tobacco when smoked increases red blood cell count and hemoglobin levels, raises immunity, increases neurotransmitter levels, enhances psychic abilities, elevates mood, and increases metabolism. In other words, it helps people think more clearly, quickly, and with less susceptibility to the establishment's control mechanisms, hence, its suppression by the establishment.

"Not everyone needs to smoke, but some <u>must</u> smoke because their genetics necessitates nicotine consumption. These are most likely ones who are already smoking and find it impossible to quit. <u>Their best alternative is to switch to pure tobacco</u>. Those without the genetic profile can nevertheless still be affected by nicotine in potentially positive ways, but I'm certainly not encouraging anyone to start smoking, just stating my observations on the effects of nicotine.

"Pure tobacco can be purchased in tobacco shops. 'American Spirit' company sells both regular pure tobacco, and organic pure tobacco. The latter is ideal. The company says that "additive-free" does not mean a safer cigarette, but you do the math. It is easy to roll cigarettes with a cheap thumb roller, or else a machine can be purchased that rolls it into tubes pre-fitted with cotton filters. Filterless cigarettes aren't truly filterless because the tobacco at one end acts as a filter - though if one prefers, cotton filter plugs can be purchased or even made from surgical cotton wool to trap larger soot particles. Because cotton is biodegradable, it does not have the same dangers as commercial cellulose acetate filters. And because such tobacco has no additives, there are fewer binders in the smoke that help tar and ash bind with lung tissue; hence it does not leave a heavy residue like commercial tobacco does.

"Of course, with a wholesome diet and healthy brain, tobacco might not be necessary unless one has a genetic need for nicotine, but it does remain as an option for anyone else willing to try it and test its supposed "performance enhancing" qualities. Clearly, the Native Americans smoked it for a time-tested reason. Unlike marijuana, pure tobacco does not interfere with willpower or mental coherence.

"While I won't necessarily recommend smoking pure tobacco to nonsmokers, I do think that those who are smoking commercial cigarettes should switch to pure tobacco as soon as possible. There is no reason to continue disposing industrial wastes via your lungs. Those with a genetic need to smoke would find it far more detrimental to quit than to continue smoking, such detriments including weight gain, immune depression, psychological depression, and mind muddling -- and what better way to continue than with a better alternative?

"For those who never want to smoke, let this commentary simply be an informative one that reveals yet another facet of the establishment's grand Agenda to manipulate and suppress mankind."

I will add only a few comments to this excellent dissertation, only to reinforce it and to add two important alternatives. Read about the benefits of the water pipe elsewhere in this book. Even taking the most noxious cigarette tobacco and smoking it through a water pipe will give you an effective, safe, and pleasurable way to get your ration of health-giving nicotine. Yes, you can inhale it. It is the only form of smoke I can recommend inhaling.

The other recommendation I have, no surprise coming from this book, is that you smoke good quality cigars, three a day – but don't inhale, except for the side stream smoke that you have created from smoking. That smoke is very diluted and almost as good as a water pipe.

Ref: Developing Ideas "http://www.montalk.net/ideas.html" http://www.montalk.net/ideas.html 6/10/03.

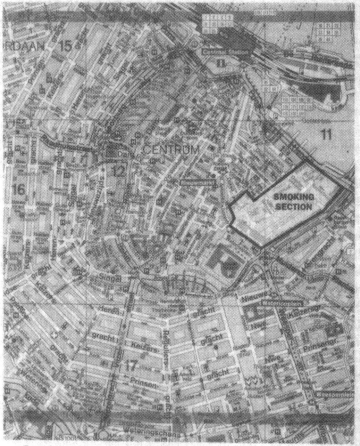

CHAPTER 25
<u>Schneiderman vs the NCI</u>

The following report by Dr. Mark Schneiderman is a response to the attempt by the National Cancer Institute to implicate cigar smoking as a causative factor in cancer and cardiovascular disease. Their dissertation is sophistic, contradictory, and obfuscatory. Dr. Schneiderman is more even-tempered than I am, and so as not to confuse his remarks with mine, my additions are in brackets and in bold face. Any emphases in Dr. Schneiderman's writings were added by me – Dr. Douglass.

A Response to the NCI Report - *Cigars: Health Effects and Trends*

Copyright 1998 by Marc J.Schneiderman, M.D.
and the Internet Cigar Group

The National Cancer Institute's (NCI) monograph <u>Cigars: Health Effects and Trends</u> was published in February, 1998. This 232 page compilation of research on the health effects of cigars is important reading for cigar smokers although <u>many conclusions are made that are often unsubstantiated by the research presented</u>. Selective research, supporting their viewpoints are offered whereas <u>debate on controversial statements is rarely presented</u>. The message the NCI wants to get out is quoted from the study below:

"Cigar smoking can cause oral, esophageal, laryngeal, and lung cancers. Regular cigar smokers who inhale, particularly those who smoke several cigars per day, have an increased risk of coronary heart disease and chronic obstructive pulmonary disease."

Regular cigar smokers have risks of oral and esophageal cancers similar to those of cigarette smokers, but they have lower risks of lung and laryngeal cancer, coronary artery disease, and chronic obstructive pulmonary disease. We believe an accurate statement is that the risks of tobacco smoke exposure are similar for all sources of tobacco smoke, and the magnitude of the risks experienced by cigar smokers is proportionate to the nature and intensity of their exposure.

(This is false as there is no evidence that there is a risk of cancer in any form from smoking cigars in moderation and in a traditional manner)

This paper attempts to summarize some of the vital topics of interest to cigar smokers from the NCI study. Many conclusions from the study can be contested and alternatives to some of these addressed.

Overview of Cigar/Disease Risks

The great majority of cigar smokers, smoke fewer than one cigar per day and don't inhale. The "habitual" cigar smoker is rarely even a daily smoker. Disease risk ratios comparing cigar smokers to the general non-smoking population are reported by NCI:

Cause of Death	Non smoker	1-2 cigars	3-4 cigars	5+ cigars
all causes	1	1. 02	1. 08	1. 17
combined oral/buccal/pharynx	1	2. 12	8. 51	15. 94
larynx cancer	1	6. 46	---	26. 03
lung cancer	1	0. 99	2. 36	2. 4
pancreas cancer	1	1. 18	1. 51	2. 21
emphysema	1	1. 39	1. 78	1. 03
coronary artery disease	1	0. 98	1. 06	1. 14

This chart demonstrates that the 1-2 cigar per day user who doesn't inhale is not at serious risk for developing cancer or heart disease. The "all cause" of death risk for smokers of 1-2 cigars per day (and sometimes more) is not significantly different when compared to those who never smoked.

The statistics presented here indicate that only cancers of the mouth and throat reveal any significance at all. Lung cancer, emphysema, and heart disease show no statistical relationship to cigar smoking. In 40 years of practice, I never saw a case of mouth or throat cancer in a patient who smoked. (That does not mean that a smoker cannot get throat cancer, unless smoke has a protective effect, which is not as outrageous as it sounds.) I had a long-time friend (50 years) who never smoked anything but he died of throat cancer. Remember that if he had ever smoked, it would have been put down as a smoking-related death. But you can rest assured his death certificate did not state: "Cause of death, cancer of the throat, never smoked." They don't keep statistics on that!

Oral cancer studies overwhelmingly suggest that the combination of cigars along with heavy alcohol use dramatically increases these cancers. Alcohol, however, was not addressed as a risk factor in the NCI report. Pancreatic cancers also are associated with alcohol. A recent study was presented demonstrating the relationship between cigar use and pancreas cancer *(Muscat, J. E.et al. , Smoking and Pancreatic Cancer in Men and Women, Cancer Epidemiology, Biomarkers, and Prevention, 6:15-19, 1997.)* One major flaw of the study is that although patients were asked about alcohol consumption, the authors did not report its effect on the pancreatic cancer results. Alcohol is a known carcinogen of the oral, pharyngeal, and GI tract (including stomach, liver, and pancreas.) Why didn't the authors comment on alcohol's impact on this group of patients with pancreatic cancer?

The NCI reports the risk ratio of cigar smokers who develop pancreatic cancer compared to the non-smoking population as 1. 18 (1-2 cigars/day.) This risk ratio is not terribly significant yet they conclude, "Cigar smokers have higher rates of pancreatic cancer than nonsmokers, particularly those who smoke higher number of cigars per day. Regression analysis confirms significant relationships with the factors of age, inhalation and cigars per day for primary cigar smokers. These data suggest that cigar smoking is a cause of pancreatic cancer." **(This is <u>a bald-faced lie</u> as their statistics show a risk ratio of 1.18, which is of <u>no statistical significance</u>.)**

They continue:" The relationship of cigar smoking and alcohol consumption, particularly for oral cancers, has not been evaluated; but the established interaction between cigarette smoking and alcohol consumption for oral cancers and the frequent association of cigar smoking with alcohol consumption raise the question of an increased risk from the combination fo (sic) these two behaviors." Although they concede a link between some cancers, tobacco and alcohol consumption, by suggesting the relationship has "not been evaluated", it weakens the argument. The studies they fail to highlight that suggest a significant positive risk between oral cancers and alcohol and tobacco are: *Wynder, 1977;Sorall, 1995; and Franceschi, 1992.*

A causal relationship between lung cancer and primary cigar smoking has been demonstrated in numerous studies (*Wynder, 1972;Gsell, 1972; Wynder,*

1977; Joly, 1983;Lublin, 1982; and Higgins, 1988.) To a large degree this relationship is influenced by inhalation practices and quantity of cigars smoked. The NCI reports that at 1-2 cigars per day, there is a lower overall risk of developing lung cancer compared to the non-smoking population (0. 99 relative risk.) Since the overwhelming majority of cigar smokers smoke fewer than 1 cigar a day and don't inhale, the majority of cigar smokers appear to be protected from developing lung cancer.

The same conclusion might be true for the risk of developing coronary artery disease in primary cigar smokers. According to the NCI, for primary cigar smokers smoking 1-2 cigars per day the incidence of coronary artery disease <u>is lower</u> than the non-smoking population (0. 98 relative risk.) Even at 5+ cigars per day the risk of coronary artery disease in this group compared to the non-smoking population is only 1. 14. **(A statistically-insignificant risk)**

The incidence of emphysema in smokers of 1-2 cigars per day is higher than the non-smoking population according to the NCI report (1. 39 relative risk.) Yet surprisingly if you smoke 5+ cigars per day the relative risk of developing emphysema plummets to 1. 03. From these data a direct relationship between cigar smoking and emphysema cannot be drawn. However the NCI report concludes, "A more accurate statement would be that the risks experienced by cigar smokers are proportionate to their exposure to tobacco smoke." **(Does <u>low</u> exposure to tobacco smoke cause a mental disconnect? –a schizophrenia? Do these National Cancer Institute doctors have cancer of the intellect? How can two cigars a day <u>increase</u> the incidence of emphysema and five cigars a day <u>decrease</u> the inci-**

dence? And then they conclude: "...the risks experienced by cigar smokers are proportionate to their exposure to tobacco smoke.")

Laryngeal cancer has been associated with cigar smoking. As with the relationship of cigar smoking to oral cancers, however, the best study to date is from *Wynder, 1977* who links it with alcohol consumption. Quoting from Wynder, "Alcohol was included in this study as an additional risk factor... the risk for each type of cancer increases with the quantity of liquor consumed, and larger proportions of heavy drinkers (and lower proportions of nondrinkers) occur for cancers of the mouth, larynx, and esophagus than do for lung or bladder cancer... Cancer of the larynx and upper alimentary tract is affected by heavy alcohol intake, as was clearly shown once more by the present study. Alcohol, whose effects interact with cigarette smoke, may be regarded as a promoter of tobacco carcinogenesis... **(That is pure supposition, based on nothing.)** Reduction of excessive alcohol consumption will have an important impact on reducing these types of cancers." *Franceschi (1992)* concurs, "Although an association could be made between cigars and oral cancer, that association based upon these numbers is not a strong one. The concurrent use of alcohol in these cancers continues to be a significant risk factor."

Their overall conclusion from the NCI about the relationship between cigar smoking and cancer, heart disease, and lung disease is as follows:

"Cigar smoking can cause oral, esophageal, laryngeal and lung cancers. Regular cigar smokers who inhale, particularly those who smoke several cigars per day, have an increased risk of coronary heart disease and chronic obstructive pulmonary disease."

My conclusions based on the NCI reported numbers and a review of the literature follow:

"Cigar smoking can cause oral, esophageal, laryngeal, and lung cancers. Still the relationship between cigar smoking and these cancers must be looked at along with other risk factors such as inhalation practices, types of cigars used, alcohol consumption, family history, and other environmental carcinogens. Studies to date do not imply a relationship between cigars and cancers of the prostate, colon, pancreas, kidneys, bone, eye, or brain."

The relationship between the development of coronary artery disease and cigar smoking has been studied. But for the non-inhaling cigar smoker who has never smoked cigarettes, and smokes 1-2 cigars per day, there is no clear-cut relationship. <u>These smokers may have lower incidences of coronary artery disease than the non-smoking population</u>. Other factors such as cigarette tobacco exposure, family history, serum cholesterol levels, hypertension, diabetes, and previous coronary events must be factored into the general risk equation.

The risk of developing emphysema has been studied in primary cigar smokers. There is a slight risk of developing this disease in the 1-2 cigar a day smoker (1. 39 relative risk) **(This statistically means <u>no risk</u>.)** As cigar consumption increases past 5 a day, however, this relative risk diminishes to approximately the same as the non-smoking population (1. 03.) These data suggest more studies are needed to investigate the relationship between emphysema and cigar smoking. Other risk factors etiological in the development of emphysema such as exposure to cigarette tobacco smoke, family history, other lung diseases and environmental contributors must be addressed in anyone considering cigar smoking.

Nicotine Dependence and Cigars

The NCI reports that cigar smoke contains many carcinogens as well as significant amounts of nicotine. "During curing and fermentation of air-cured tobacco, nitrate is partially reduced to nitrite, most likely by microbal (sic) action. This contributes to the N-nitrosation of nicotine, converting it into the highly carcinogenic, tobacco-specific N-nitrosamines (TSNA), N-nitrosonornicotine (NNN) and 4-(methylnitrosamino)-1-(3-pyridyl)-1-butanone (NNK) *(Burton et al. , 1992; Hoffmann et al. , 1994;Wiernik et al. , 1995)*. . . . *Rickert et al.(1985)* examined the delivery of 'tar,' nicotine and CO per liter of smoke for different tobacco products. They found that the mean yields per liter of smoke were highest for small cigars followed by hand-rolled and manufactured cigarettes and were lowest for large cigars. Total delivery was greatest for large cigars because of their larger amount of tobacco . . .. Carbon monoxide and nicotine are major contributors to the acute toxicity of cigar smoke. Among agents which also add to the acute toxicity of cigar smoke are nitrogen oxides, hydrogen cyanide, ammonia, and volatile aldehydes." **(Small amounts of carbon monoxide and nicotine are good for your health, especially your cardiovascular health.)**

Do cigar smokers absorb nicotine and carbon monoxide? Clearly these agents factor into the development of coronary artery disease. The NCI data demonstrates that primary cigar smokers do not develop coronary artery disease more frequently compared to the non-smoking population if they smoke 1-2 cigars per day. This suggests that either cigar nicotine is not easily absorbed through the oral mucosa (carbon monoxide is only absorbed through the lung) or the amount of second hand smoke that non-inhalers are exposed to is minimal.

The conclusions of the NCI are that:

- Cigar smoke contains the same toxic and carcinogenic compounds identified in cigarette smoke.

- The amount of nicotine available as free, unprotonated nicotine is generally higher in cigars than in cigarettes due to the higher pH of cigar smoke. This free nicotine is readily absorbed across the oral mucosa, and may explain why cigar smokers are less likely to inhale than cigarette smokers.

The NCI reports that two studies are conclusive that nicotine is absorbed orally and cigar smokers get a nicotine "hit" without inhaling. One study from 1970 (*Armitage and D. M.Turner, Absorption of Nicotine in Cigarette and Cigars Smoke through the Oral Mucosa, Nature, 226:1231-1232*) studied cats blood pressure and ear twitching response to smoke (cigar and cigarette) installed into their mouths while anesthetized. Cigar smoke elevated their blood pressure but cigarette smoke did not. No controls were used. The conclusion of this "study" was that, "The present evidence indicates that cigarette smokers who do not inhale may not obtain a 'stimulant' dose of nicotine from relatively acidic smoke. It may, however, be possible for a cigars smoker to obtain such a dose without inhaling."

<u>There were obvious flaws in this study</u>: (1) no correlation of blood levels of nicotine with a physiologic response; (2) lack of controls; (3) the effect of inhaling a more irritating alkaline smoke (cigars) to the more acidic, but less irritating smoke (cigarettes). **(You would have to be <u>crazy</u> to inhale cigar smoke.)** Basing conclusions on better studies comparing serum nicotine and carboxyhemoglobin (reflective of carbon monoxide exposure) levels of cigarette smokers and cigar smokers would have been more appropriate. **(Dr. Schneiderman is too kind. This sophomoric study would not make a "D" in a high school biology class.)**

Armitage et al. attempted this study, (*Armitage, et al. , Absorption of nicotine from small cigars. Clinical Pharmacology and Therapeutics, 23(2): 143-151.*)

The NCI concludes from this study that cigar smokers absorb nicotine. Male current habitual cigarette smokers, who were told not to smoke after midnight the night before the experiment began, were used for this study. The volunteers then smoked small cigars and arterial blood was evaluated at 10-minute intervals for nicotine and carbon monoxide levels. They were categorized as either "inhaler" or "slight inhaler/nonsmoker". Cigars and cigarettes were compared. The authors conclude that "Buccal absorption of nicotine is slower and less complete than absorption by the alveolar capillaries ... We conclude that cigar smokers can achieve plasma nicotine concentrations as high as those in cigarette smokers by a variable combination of inhalation into the alveoli and mucosal absorption. As the rate of rise of plasma nicotine is slower in cigar smokers, the short-term pharmacologic effects are likely to be less than those in cigarette smokers since the principal pharmacologic effects of nicotine relate not so much to the blood concentration achieved but to the rate of change in that concentration. This probably explains why the heart rate changes observed during cigar smoking were less than after cigarette smoking."

The obvious flaw of this study is in using cigarette-starved "current and habitual" cigarette smokers to smoke small cigars. There is no question that these volunteers would inhale a good deal of smoke. Numerous studies demonstrate that ex-cigarette smokers who smoke cigars inhale them (even though they report they don't). It would have been more appropriate to compare the nicotine levels of current "habitual" primary cigar smokers (who never smoked cigarettes) to cigarette smokers.

There is a study that did just that.(*Turner, et al. , Effect of cigar smoking on carboxyhemoglobin and plasma nicotine concentrations in primary pipe and cigar smokers and ex-cigarette smokers. British Medical Journal 2: 1387-1389, 1977.*) Surprisingly primary cigar smokers DID NOT develop the same serum nicotine or carboxyhemoglobin levels as cigarette smokers. Blood levels of nicotine and carboxyhemoglobin in primary cigar smokers were comparable to those who were exposed only to second hand smoke. [Which, as you will see, if you read this entire book, is of no consequence. However, ex-cigarette smokers who were smoking cigars did develop the nicotine and carboxyhemoglobin levels of current cigarette smokers.

Recall that carbon monoxide is only absorbed through the lungs. Also, serum carboxyhemoglobin levels accurately reflect exposure to carbon monoxide. Given the elevated serum carboxyhemoglobin levels demonstrated in ex-cigarette smokers who smoke cigars, it is clear that ex-cigarette smokers, even though they report no inhalation, do inhale.

The authors conclude, "Since ex-cigarette smokers do not seem to lose their habit of inhaling when they change to cigars, measures aimed at persuading smokers to switch to cigars will have little effect on their health. Pipe and cigar smokers who have never smoked cigarettes do not inhale, which probably accounts for their reduced incidence of coronary heart disease and lung cancer. But they also appear not to absorb nicotine, which suggests that nicotine is absorbed largely from the lung and that the buccal mucosa is unimportant. It also raises the interesting question of why primary pipe and cigars smokers do smoke." The authors could easily answer that last "interesting question" by lighting up a fine Havana.

The NCI study further concludes "There is sufficient nicotine absorption among regular heavy cigar smokers to expect that nicotine dependence might develop, but studies to document the frequency or intensity of nicotine dependence have not been published."

It's not a mistake to state that for the great majority of primary cigar smokers, addiction to cigars is not an issue. Most cigar smokers smoke less than one a day and habitual cigar smokers do not appear to increase their consumption over time. By the way, ever see a group of cigar smokers standing outside a smoke-free office building in the middle of winter to get a cigar "hit"? Unlike cigarette studies, there are no reports demonstrating that teenage cigar users continue smoking cigars into adulthood. Teenage cigarette addiction however is well documented. NCI admits that, "The extensive studies of time course and symptomology of withdrawal symptoms that have been conducted in cigarette smokers have not been duplicated in cigar smokers." Still they go on to conclude, "several lines of evidence suggests that it may be possible cigar smokers to develop a similar syndrome of withdrawal." **(Show us the proof)**.

The NCI concludes that since nicotine is addicting, absorption through the oral mucosa, is present in cigars, and studies (Armitage) demonstrate nicotine absorption via cigar smoking, then obviously nicotine addiction would follow, along with typical withdrawal symptoms. It is also clear that cigar smokers are not addicted in the same way as cigarette smokers. NCI tries to explain this: "Lower rates of inhalation in cigar smokers and slower absorption of nicotine through the buccal mucosa suggest that cigar smoking may have a lower potential to induce addiction to nicotine than cigarette smoking. In addition, it is plausible that persons who never had been nicotine dependent and who began smoking cigars in adulthood would be at a lower risk for developing dependence than children and adolescents who take up tobacco use. It does appear that a much higher proportion of adult cigar users compared to adult cigarette smokers are non-daily users."

Nicotine is more addicting in children than adults? This type of statement, which cannot be substantiated, and doesn't even sound plausible, is present throughout the NCI monograph. Another example can be found in the discussion about why cigar smokers don't inhale." While almost all cigarette smokers inhale, the majority of cigar smokers do not. This may be due to differences in the pH of the smoke produced by these two products. Cigar smoke contains a substantial fraction of its nicotine as free nicotine, which can be readily absorbed across the oral mucosa. In contrast, cigarette smoke is more acidic, and the protonated form of nicotine it contains is much less readily absorbed by the oral mucosa. As a result, cigarette smokers must inhale to get their required quantity of nicotine, whereas cigar smokers can ingest sufficient quantities of nicotine without inhaling." <u>Turner effectively demonstrated that primary cigar smokers do not develop serum levels of nicotine above those exposed only to second hand smoke</u>. **(Which is minute and therefore of no health significance.)** And, if ex-cigarette smokers who currently smoke cigars could get their "required quantity of nicotine" via the oral route, why then do they need to inhale?

Some Final Thoughts

In summary the NCI report sheds little new light on the issues of the health effects of cigars. It is at best an excellent compilation of the research to date. The report reminds us that today adolescents in increasing numbers are experimenting with cigars. Major cigar publications, organizations, and personalities, have publicly denounced any tobacco use by adolescents. The decision to responsibly use cigars in moderation is a decision to be made by adults. Responsible use dictates limiting the number of cigars smoked and non inhaling.

My recommendation is that ex-cigarette users refrain from taking up cigars as an alternative to cigarettes and heavy alcohol users should stay away from any tobacco product. Finally, all risk factors for cancer, lung and heart disease, i.e. cigarette smoking, family history, serum cholesterol levels, concurrent high risk diseases (diabetes, hypertension, asthma, etc.) and lifestyle (diet, exercise) must be evaluated in each individual undertaking cigar smoking. Cigar smoking is not without risk but I believe the NCI report clearly demonstrates that those risks are acceptable to those who use the product responsibly.

See Appendix: From the Cigar Baron

Ref: Marc J. Schneiderman, M.D. garbaron@telerama.lm.com

SECTION VI
APPENDIX

APPENDIX A

<u>HEART</u>

A Contrary Study Without Merit

In this study, we examined the impact of **smoking** on both clinical and angiographic outcomes of contemporary PCI, including balloon angioplasty, directional atherectomy, and coronary stenting. Our major finding was that although smokers experienced a 31% reduction in clinical restenosis (ie, TLR), paradoxically there were no differences in angiographic restenosis or other angiographic parameters at follow-up according to **smoking** status. Although there were important differences in baseline clinical and angiographic characteristics between smokers and nonsmokers, our findings persisted in multivariable analyses that controlled for these differences.

Comparison With Previous Studies

To date, Hasdai and colleaguesp://circ.ahajournals.org/cgi/content/full/104/7/" \l "R2-094225" \o "http://circ.ahajournals.org/cgi/content/full/104/7/#R2-094225" [2] have performed the largest study of the impact of smoking on the outcomes of PCI. In their cohort of >5400 patients, they found that compared with nonsmokers, former smokers and persistent smokers had a 20% and 33% reduction, respectively, in the need for repeated revascularization during the first year of follow-up—results remarkably similar to our experience. However, their study lacked systematic angiographic follow-up in a subset of patients and was thus unable to elucidate the precise mechanism for this apparent "benefit" of smoking. Other studies that have examined the impact of smoking on angiographic restenosis have generally found no differences in either angiographic or clinical outcomes between smokers and nonsmokers.\l "R3-094225" \o "http://circ.ahajournals.org/cgi/content/full/104/7/#R3-094225" [3]\l "R4-094225" \o "http://circ.ahajournals.org/cgi/content/full/104/7/#R4-094225"[4] However, the performance of angiographic follow-up in the full population of these studies limited their ability to reliably assess clinical outcomes because of the well-recognized oculostenotic reflex.\l "R6-094225" \o "http://circ.ahajournals.org/cgi/content/full/104/7/#R6-094225" [6] Until now, it has been unclear whether these differences between angiographic and clinical outcomes reflect underlying differences in the patient populations of the various studies or a true case of "angiographic-clinical dissociation.". ahajournals.org/cgi/content/full/104/7/" \l "R16-094225" \o "http://circ.ahajournals.org/cgi/content/full/104/7/#R16-094225" [16] By virtue of its split-sample design and large sample size, our study is the first to definitively demonstrate that the reduction in clinical restenosis associated with smoking is not due to a reduction in angiographic restenosis. Moreover, our study extends the results of previous studies by demonstrating these findings in a group of patients undergoing contemporary PCI (mainly coronary stenting).

Cardiovascular Disease and Infection

From Chapter 242 Harrison's Textbook of Medicine

<u>Prevention and Treatment of Atherosclerosis</u>
<u>Infection/Inflammation</u>

Recent years have witnessed a resurgence of interest in the possibility that infections may cause or contribute to atherosclerosis. A spate of recent publications has furnished evidence in support for a role of *Chlamydia pneumoniae*, cytomegalovirus, or other infectious agents in atherosclerosis and restenosis following coronary intervention. Some microorganisms exist in human atherosclerotic plaques. However, seroepidemiologic evidence for an association between infection with various agents and atherosclerosis remains inconclusive. Several ongoing large trials of antibiotic treatment in survivors of myocardial infarction may provide support for an etiologic or contributory role of microbial infection in recurrent coronary events. Even if positive, however, such clinical trials would neither inculpate any particular microorganisms nor even prove that a benefit derived from the antimicrobial action of the agent employed.

Although direct infection may not cause atherosclerosis, the infectious agents and the host defenses against these invaders might potentiate atherogenesis, acting as inflammatory stimuli. Just as inflammation may mediate some of the altered arterial biology in response to hyperlipoproteinemia, so might infectious agents incite an inflammatory response that could promote atherosclerosis and its complications. Thus, microbial pathogens might act in concert with traditional risk factors to accelerate atherogenesis or cause complication or aggravation of existing atheroma.

In this regard, evidence is accumulating that markers of inflammation correlate with coronary risk. For example, elevated plasma levels of C-reactive protein (CRP) can prospectively predict risk of myocardial infarction and correlate with outcome of patients with acute coronary syndromes. As in the case of fibrinogen, elevated levels of the acute-phase reactant CRP may merely reflect ongoing inflammation rather than a direct etiologic role for CRP in coronary artery disease. It remains uncertain whether elevations in acute-phase reactants such as fibrinogen or CRP serve as a marker for the overall atherosclerotic burden, and hence of coronary events. Alternatively, the elevation in acute-phase reactants could reflect extravascular inflammation that could potentiate atherosclerosis or its complications. In all likelihood, both factors contribute to elevation of inflammatory markers in patients at risk for coronary events. These observations raise the possibility that anti-inflammatory therapies might reduce atherosclerotic events. Indeed, lipid-lowering therapy may reduce coronary events in part by reducing the inflammatory aspects of the pathogenesis of atherosclerosis.

Monica Project

BMJ   1998;317:1023   (10 October)
Views and reviews
Medicine and the media

Did MONICA really say that?

Can I have a fag and a chip butty now? Some journalists have claimed, on the basis of the results of the MONICA project, those coronary risk factors no longer matter. Hugh Tunstall-Pedoe, who was involved in the study, explains how the media metamorphosed the original story.

Americans' inability to explain their decline in coronary disease spawned the World Health Organization's MONICA project (MONItoring CArdiovascular disease) in the 1980s. This 10-year study of trends in disease and risk factors recruited 38 populations in 21 countries. Preliminary results were presented at the European Congress of Cardiology in Vienna in August 1998 but individual centers had previously published results.

I drafted the press release accompanying this presentation; it emphasized the value of the data on trends collected from the 38 populations and listed findings for coronary disease rates, 28 day case fatality, smoking, blood pressure, cholesterol, and obesity. Then came the surprises. Although some centers had previously reported no change in case fatality during the revolution in treatment of myocardial infarction of the 1980s, scatter plots showed an unexpectedly strong relation between trends in treatment and in case fatality and also in mortality and event rates.

Contrariwise, North Karelia and Iceland had reported (in the *BMJ*) good relations between their decline in coronary disease rates and in risk factors. The scatter plots of the 38 centersshowed an unexpectedly weak relation between the size of the decline in disease rates and in individual risk factors, and in a composite risk factor score. There were possible technical explanations. How much the conventional risk factors might explain awaited further analyses. Meanwhile there was room for extraneous factors, which MONICA was not equipped to identify.

Both the press release and press conference emphasized that the importance of conventional risk factors had been shown by innumerable observational and interventional studies, more powerful than MONICA through being based on individuals. Advice to the individual was therefore not affected.

But then came the media reports. "Study casts doubt on heart `risk factors'" was the headline in the *Daily Telegraph* on 25 August. "The largest ever cardiology study has failed to find a link between heart attacks and the classic risk factors, such as smoking and high cholesterol levels." Later paragraphs were more faithful to the press release, but a quotation from me was followed, as if from me, by the presumption that stress was the missing factor. Still in Vienna, I participated by hotel room telephone in a chat show on BBC Radio 2. I told the researcher to discount what was written in the *Daily Telegraph* and use our press release. But still the interviewer said: "There is no connection between heart disease and smoking, blood pressure, or cholesterol." I denied it and tried to explain. "It is all caused by stress," the interviewer said. (At this point the elderly chambermaid marched in regardless and thumped about in the bathroom.) I denied it. "You said that in the *Daily Telegraph*." I denied it. "Really, we know nothing at all about what causes heart disease." I denied it and tried to summarize 50 years of cardiovascular epidemiology in a few pithy sentences. The interview terminated with a curt "Thank YOU." I could imagine faces being pulled.

A freelance journalist wrote up the story carefully for the *Independent* health page (1 September) with a low nonsense quotient. Two weeks later (15 September) another journalist had a go in the same column. "Doctor, doctor—can I have a fag and a chip butty now? After 20 years of scolding us about tobacco and cholesterol, experts have had their come-uppance. The world's largest and longest study of heart disease... has shown that these risk factors are apparently irrelevant." The *Independent* published replies from the British Heart Foundation and myself two days later. Finally BBC Radio Scotland requested discussion on its Saturday morning *Newsweek* programme. Again, despite its access to our press release, I was challenged with the newspaper headlines and offered little time to reply. A discussant said that some risk stories were based on phony statistics, so the interviewer suggested that this included coronary risk factors and MONICA. After minimal discussion the interview ended; I was offered a fee.

Having myself insisted that a prepared press release would minimize media distortion, I find my MONICA colleagues aghast at the British press. The headlines are now spreading out around the world from Britain. Journalists prefer quoting each other's headlines to checking their sources. Even colleagues quote the headlines accusingly. As in politics, denial is taken to mean the story is true. Little now separates the tabloid press and other media.

Non-numeracy undoubtedly contributes. Papers that headline "Prices fall" when inflation comes down show their inability to distinguish a factor from its differential. Journalists are not alone in mistakenly believing that prevention demands complete knowledge of causal factors. If causation is conceptually additive, then unknown factors diminish the significance of known ones. But coronary risk is multiplicative. Stopping smoking halves your risk regardless of the number of other factors, known or unknown. Try explaining that.

There is a chasm between what MONICA said and what the media said she said, but most people get their information from the media.

Hugh Tunstall-Pedoe.

Cardiovascular Epidemiology Unit, Ninewells Hospital and Medical School, Dundee DD1 9SY

The Real Causes of Heart Disease

The Seven Countries Study

Fifty-two years ago, the Ancel Keys Seven Countries Study showed that there was no relation between smoking and heart disease.

The anti-smoking demagogues have produced an endless stream of deceitful and misleading statements on smoking, side stream smoke and heart disease. It has been known since the Seven Countries studies of the 1960s that smoking rates do not correlate with the wide variations in heart disease rates between different countries. From the Keys report:

> "Differences in the all-causes mortality or coronary death rate or the coronary incidence rates of the cohorts could not be shown to be related to any measure of the smoking habits of the cohorts -- the proportion of the men who were nonsmokers, the proportion who were heavy smokers, the average cigarettes per day, and so on." (Seven Countries: A

multivariate analysis of death and coronary heart disease, by Ancel Keys, p. 325).

There were some "puzzling" and "paradoxical' findings in the Keys report. Some countries had high rates of smoking and that country's nonsmokers had lower rates of heart disease. Well, OK – just as the anti-smokers would like it. It means that smoking causes heart disease – right? Well now for the "paradox," – smokers in countries with low rates of heart disease <u>have lower rates of heart disease than non-smokers in countries with high rates</u>. That's a little confusing but the bottom line is: there is no plausible relationship between smoking and heart disease. Although Dr. Howard is throwing kitchen sinks at the facts, the facts will not change.

Smokers in countries with low rates of cardiovascular disease <u>have lower rates than non-smokers in countries with high rates</u>. Therefore, the study's lead off claim that "Smoking is a powerful risk factor for incident heart disease and stroke," when it does not account for those differences, is an outright lie as well.

Thanks to recent research, we now know that those varying rates of heart disease in different countries <u>DO correlate with plasma homocysteine levels</u> (*Plasma homocysteine and cardiovascular disease mortality.* G Alfthan, A Aro, KF Gey. The Lancet 1997 Feb 8;349:397). But this study, as well as the accompanying editorial, <u>fail to mention homocysteine</u> even once.

And when the health establishment does mention it, they try to trump up the supposed role of smoking instead; by admitting only that homocysteine might play "perhaps as large a role as smoking," (Newsweek 1997 August 11, "The Heart Attackers," by Geoffrey

Cowley). <u>Yet homocysteine accounts for drastic differences in cardiovascular disease rates, while smoking does not</u>.

This study and the editorial also fail to mention Helicobacter pylori and Chlamydia pneumoniae infection, which many studies have linked to cardiovascular disease. Nor is there mention of C-reactive protein, a general marker of inflammation. These anti-smoker bunko artists and their media confederates just brazenly ignore these important risk factors, and base their hysterical accusations on defective studies with incomplete, inadequate, and out-of-date selections of risk factors, and misrepresent them as complete.

It is known that HP infection occurs in early childhood, before smoking begins, and therefore infection at older ages is extremely rare. The infection persists throughout life, unless treated by a unique combination of drugs. There may also be a link between Helicobacter pylori, homocysteine and heart disease, in that patients with HP-caused gastritis suffer malabsorption of cobalamin, an essential cofactor for methionine synthetase.

HP infection is more common in the lower socioeconomic classes, and in blacks, as is smoking, and HP is more common among both smokers and passive smokers, who share smokers' socioeconomic characteristics. <u>Because of this, the anti-smokers have blamed smoking for heart disease caused by HP.</u>

In this study, the socioeconomic and racial differences by smoking and ETS status are clearly shown by the proxy variable of educational level. It compares a group more likely to be white female college graduate not exposed never smokers, versus white male college grad not exposed ex-smokers, versus current smokers who are more likely than the former to be black high school dropouts. By ETS exposure, groups most likely to be college grads are compared with groups most likely to be high school grads.

Howard et al. admitted that the socioeconomic differences were "dramatic." Those differences were supposedly adjusted for, but the use of proxy variables instead of true risk factors is known to be insufficient to control for the effect of true risks, and often false ones are implicated. Anti-smokers have pulled this trick on us before to blame smoking for ulcers actually caused by HP, so there is no reason to trust them.

In fact, the raw average progression was the same between smokers and ETS-exposed never or ex-smokers (37 fm), who also shared the characteristic of most likely being high school grads, nor was it much different between non-exposed never or ex-smokers (31 & 32 fm), who shared the characteristic of most likely being college grads.

The ostensible differences within those educational groupings, which they attributed to smoke exposure, were entirely artificially produced. So it is far more accurate to say that Howard et al. threw the kitchen sink at the data to fabricate those claims, not to make them go away. Isn't epidemiology a marvelous science?

Chlamydia pneumoniae infection has been linked to atherosclerosis, heart attack and stroke. Even the AHA has been forced to grudgingly acknowledge the evidence (Press release. <u>American Heart Association's Top Research Advances....</u> U.S. Newswire OTC 12/31 1410). Gupta showed that heart attack patients with high antibody levels to CP who were given antibiotics had no more risk of a second heart attack than uninfected patients (Gupta S et al. Elevated Chlamydia pneumoniae antibodies, cardiovascular events, and azithromycin in male survivors of myocardial infarction. Circulation 1997 Jul 15; 96(2): 404-407).

The media embellished this story with an anti-smoker mouthpiece, Dr. Valentin Fuster, who was not even associated with Gupta's study, to dissemble to us that "It is possible," he said, "that further study could show that the bacterium is as important a trigger for heart attacks as cigarette smoking," to encourage the false belief that it is not necessary to inquire whether CP is actually responsible for supposed smoking risks (Infection May Predict Heart Attack. AP 15-Jul-1997 10:30 EDT REF5251).

Regarding Howard, The AP told us, "Dr. Stanton A. Glantz, a secondhand smoke expert at the University of California-San Francisco, said the study `provides a real important bridge' between studies that have found that cigarette smoke causes deteriorating arteries and studies showing that passive smokers have an increased risk of fatal heart attacks. `This fills in that missing link,' Glantz said." Except that all of those studies committed the same epidemiologic malpractice.

Glantz's claim to fame is his trumpeting of animal studies of ETS exposure and atherosclerosis. These studies induced atherosclerosis with unnatural high-fat diets, and then contended that there was a statistically significant difference between the exposed and non-exposed. We are expected to consider these as conclusive as an animal study showing that infection with Chlamydia pneumoniae alone caused atherosclerosis, in the absence of any other risk factors (Fong IW et al. Rabbit model for Chlamydia pneumoniae infection. J Clin Microbiol 1997 Jan; 35(1): 48-52).

Glantz's speculations purporting a role for PAHs are discredited by the high levels of PAHs in food, which overwhelm any possible contribution from ETS (HA Hattemer-Frey, CC Travis. Benzo-a-pyrene: Environmental partitioning and human exposure. Toxicology and Industrial Health 1991; 7(3): 141-157).

"Previous studies have shown that secondhand smoke, like active smoking, can kill by causing more acute but reversible problems, such as thickening of the blood," the AP told us.

Except that the real cause of such "thickening of the blood" could very well be HP, CP, or other infection (IY Bova et al. Acute infection as a risk factor for ischemic stroke. Stroke 1996;27:2204-2206). And until studies properly evaluate this risk, they should desist from all such pronouncements about both secondhand smoke and active smoking.

The American Heart Association resorted to the most despicable demagoguery of all, by exploiting children: "This study provides more evidence that in order to protect the health of all non-smokers, particularly children, smoking must be banned in all public places, including restaurants" (AHA press release).

In fact, the main vectors of CP infection are children, especially ages 7-13. CP infection is particularly common in them, probably due to exposure to each other's hygiene in school. They bring the infection home to their families. This indicates that, rather than smokers causing heart disease in children, children cause heart disease in adults. And the most important public measures would be getting them to wash their hands and keep their fingers out of their noses. But the AHA couldn't care less when there are smokers to attack.

"Hardening of the arteries, or atherosclerosis, is responsible for more deaths in the United States than any other single cause," the media dutifully informed us (Knight-Ridder). So, see how the anti-smoker research establishment diverts attention and funding from investigating the real causes of disease into persecuting smoking instead.

The anti-smoker health establishment refuses to design or analyze studies to determine whether these important new risk factors explain the alleged risks of smoking. They want no data released to the public that could be usable by smoking defenders.

Then, their demagogues have the gall to <u>accuse the tobacco industry of supposedly concealing data</u>, not one example of which is ever put forth, because none exist; and of "misdirecting" research toward defending smoking, instead of witch hunting for bogus "smoking dangers" as the anti-smoking crowd prefers. If only this were true, we all would have been better off.

The tobacco industry's response is pathetic, as usual: "Tom Lauria, a spokesman for The Tobacco Institute, which is funded by the tobacco industry, said advocates there had not yet evaluated the study". But he noted: "The majority of studies do not show any increased risk for nonsmokers. We consider the science to be inconclusive" (AP). The tobacco industry has yet to utter a peep about the evidence casting doubt upon the anti-smokers' claims.

The American Heart Association chimed in on this vicious deceit. "`If a non-smoker is around a person who smokes a pack of cigarettes during the day, the non-smoker's exposure is so great that it's almost comparable to his or her smoking half of that pack of cigarettes,' said Aubrey Taylor, Ph.D., an AHA spokesperson and lead author of an American Heart Association statement on environmental tobacco smoke" (AHA press release).

In fact, the study found that "there was no evidence of a dose-response relationship between increasing weekly hours of ETS exposure and increased progression rates among those exposed to ETS" (which failed to come out in the media). This gives weight to the idea that the purported ETS risk is really due to the risk factors they left out. It also shows that the AHA feels free to dispense with the requirement for a dose-response at will.

The Journal of the American Medical Association placed its official seal of approval on scientific fraud: "Not much is passive about 'passive smoke,'" wrote the editorial authors, Rachel Werner and Dr. Thomas Pearson of the University of Rochester School of Medicine in Rochester, N.Y. "What is passive is our lack of recognition of the importance of passive smoke as a cardiovascular disease risk factor, our oversight in not asking patients about this exposure, and our lack of advocacy for clean air as a way to help prevent chronic disease," they wrote (AP). Their indifference to the real risk factors and to scientific integrity can be characterized a lot more harshly than merely "passive."

Ref: Carol Thompson 1-19-98 Smokers' Rights Action Group.
P.O.Box259575 Madison, WI 53725-9575.

It is amazing how easy it is to get people to seize upon an illogical or even preposterous idea and within a span of six weeks of relentless TV propaganda, turn the ridiculous theory into a well-known scientific fact. That is what happened with the "side stream" or "second hand," smoke hypothesis. One day it was an unknown thing and, only a few weeks later, everyone was an expert on the dire threat to pregnant mothers, babies, the elderly and – especially – neurotic women and their cohorts of the opposite sex - the pecksniff pinko boys in the environmental red brigades. This hysteria has gone so far that we now have smokeless hotels, smokeless airports, and 100 percent smokeless airlines. Smokers are the scum of the earth, putrid polluters and a threat to all mankind -- all of that in a span of 6 months!

The only other case of national, and international, hysteria that I have seen develop in an even shorter period of time was the famous Orson Wells' radio show back in the 1930s: The War of the Worlds. Mr. Wells produced a drama about the invasion of our planet by foreign humanoids. It came on during prime time radio with dramatic, minute-by-minute updates. There was panic in the streets and multiple accidents, as people sought to escape to they knew not where. In 24 hours the panic subsided as the airways were saturated with the good news that it was only a radio drama. The closest thing to this comic episode, proving the gullibility of man, is the "side stream (or "second hand") smoke" terror blitz. Even in former smoker's paradises, such as Panama and Spain, smokers are being dogged and cast out of restaurants, opulent and ordinary, in the name of stopping the cancer epidemic being perpetrated by the putrid and pathetic puffers.

On a cruise ship in the South Pacific, I experienced a pathetic, but amusing, episode in the cigar bar (Yes, they actually had one, but it's probably a non-smoking juice bar now). One had to go through the bar to go from the restaurant to the bow of the ship. Four 18ish girls went dashing through the bar at full speed with handkerchiefs over their faces.

It may give you a creepy feeling to find out that the first serious anti-smoking campaign by a government, for the health of the people of course, was the German Nazi party. Read the book, The Nazi War on Cancer. The similarities are chilling. Hitler and his propaganda minister, Joseph Goebels, used the Hitler Youth and the Green Party in an attempt to stamp out smoking. (It didn't work.)

The Nazi doctors took the lead in the fight against tobacco. They were 20 years ahead of their American counterparts who were promoting smoking and making millions through selling cigarette advertising in the medical journals. Like most everything else, it was turned into a genetic and racial issue. Cigarettes, they claimed, affected the gene pool so smoking was a threat to the purity of the race and, anyway, it was being promoted for this very purpose by Jews, Gypsies, whores, Africans and Indians. (Hitler was an equal opportunity persecutor.)

But let's not give the Nazis undue credit for their "progressive" attitude toward smoking. As far back as 1620 resistance to the evil weed was vigorous and, in 1691, persons in Luneberg caught smoking could be put to death! As today, it was the self-righteous liberals who were seized with near madness and not the smokers. A smoker, caught in the degenerate act, could be beaten, banished, jailed with forced labor, or marked with a firebrand.

One "expert" with the National Cancer Institute or the American Cancer Society (same thing) proclaims: "If you are sitting next to a smoker, you might as well be smoking yourself. Your exposure is the equivalent of smoking half a cigarette." That is a **preposterous lie** but most people believe it!

But the very same NCI, in the Journal of the National Cancer Institute published (March 1998), a World Health Organization WHO)/IARC study that found **no statistically significant increase in lung cancer risk for nonsmokers living or working with smokers**.

That opinion was unacceptable to all concerned in the smoke cover-up, the people who like to blow smoke about smoking (including the WHO). So a few years later, the Environmental Protection Agency (EPA), which is always howling after the smokers, produced an obfuscatory masterpiece that "proved" the WHO/ARC study to be wrong and without any merit whatsoever. I say "obfuscatory masterpiece" because the EPA "study" <u>wasn't a study at all</u> but simply a collection of poorly controlled secondhand smoke papers, bundled together so as to form a majority opinion; in other words, "science through democracy." In research, they call this type of often-misleading and inaccurate study a "meta analysis." It makes it sound scientific. Incidentally, not all of the papers so bundled found any risk from side stream smoke. But in this type of pseudo study, majority rules, not science.

Ref: Journal of the National Cancer Institute, 1998; 90:1440-50 London Telegraph, 3/8/98, Victoria Macdonald

They failed in their attempt to hide the results of the original study. The research was eventually published in the Journal of the National Cancer Institute (1998; 90:1440-50), but only after the London Telegraph (and the London Times) broke a story on the findings of the paper and accused WHO of suppressing the information ("Passive smoking doesn't cause cancer--official," by Victoria Macdonald, London Telegraph, 3/8/98).

The IARC study is credible because it represented the best effort of an <u>anti-tobacco</u> organization to find evidence that secondhand smoke is hazardous to human health. It attains greater credibility because it was conducted according to accepted epidemiology standards. The tobacco-control Mafia wishes this study would vanish from the face of the earth or, at the very least, be forgotten and ignored. The WHO's "new" study, which came to an opposite conclusion, was designed to neutralize the first study. With suppression of the first paper by most of the media, this was easily accomplished. Many of the same researchers were involved in BOTH reports. Yet, the conclusions were diametrically opposed to the first report.

A federal judge <u>vacated the EPA report</u> because the procedures used were not "up to snuff." Even had the report not been vacated, meta-analysis as a method of epidemiological research is almost always corrupted by personal biases.

> "There are many problems with meta-analysis as a tool. One huge problem is that those conducting the meta-analysis must be without bias. For example, they must not cherry-pick the data to include only those epidemiological studies that show the conclusions they want (remember, the federal judge said the EPA had cherry-picked the studies it used in its meta-analysis). "

Ref: Wanda Hamilton (FORCES) on meta-analysis.

But even if the meta-analyzer is honest, he or she (or they) can still come to invalid results because if some of the studies included are themselves not well designed, their results could be invalid. A meta-analysis including weak or poorly designed (or flawed) studies will itself be flawed.

Also, there is a problem if the studies do not study the same populations or include the same confounders. For example, if some studies control for age and socio-economic status and others do not, it would be like lumping apples in with oranges. The likelihood of epidemiological studies being similar enough in design to be able to lump their results together and then do some statistical manipulation to come up with a sort of "average" relative risk is VERY small.

It's bizarre in the extreme that when more than 80% of the epidemiological studies ever conducted show NO statistically significant increased risk of lung cancer in never-smokers exposed to spousal smoking, the meta-analyzers can come up with a statistically significant risk. The only way they can do that is to cherry pick the studies they include...

Ref: Journal of the National Cancer Institute, 1998;90:1440-50.

NEUROLOGICAL DISEASES

Parkinson's and Alzheimer's Disease
Studies and Publications

Amaducci LA, et al. A case-controlled study of an Italian population. *Neurology*, 1986, 36:922-931.

Barclay L, Kheyfets S. Tobacco used in Alzeimer's disease. *Prog. Clin. Bho. Res* 0989, 317:189-194.

Brenner DE, et al. Relationship between cig. smoking and Alz. disease. *Neurology* 1993, 43:293-300.

Broe GA et al. A case -controlled study of alz. in Australia. *Neurology* 1990, 40:1698-1707.

Chandra V. et al. Case study of the late on-set 'probable Alz. disease'. *Neurology* 1987, 37:1295-1300.

Dewey ME, et al. Risk factors for Dementia. Liverpool, Int. *Geriatric Psychiatry* 1988, 3:245-249.

Ferini-Strambi, et al. Clinical Aspect of Alz. Disease with pre-senile on-set. *Neuro Epidem* 1990, 9:34-49.   French LR, et al. Case-control study of dementia of Alz. type. *Am J Epidemiol* 1985, 121:414-421.

Graves, AB, et al. Case controlled study of Alz. disease. *Neurol* 1990, 28:766-774.

Grossberg, GT, et al. Smoking as a risk factor for Alz disease. *Am. Geriatric Soc.* 1989, 37:819.

Hebert LE, et al. Relation of smoking and alcohol to Alz disease. *Amer. J Epidemiol* 1992, 135:347-355.

Heyman A, et al. Alz disease: a study of epidem aspects. *Am Neurol* 1984, 15:335-341.

Hofman A, van Duijn. Alz disease, Parkinson's disease, and smoking. *Neurobiol Aging* 1990, 11:295.

Jones GMM, et al. Smoking and dementia of Alz type. *Neurol Neurosurg Psychiatry* 1987, 50:1383.

Joya CJ, et al. Risk factors in clinically-diagnosed Alz disease. *SA Neuroniol Aging* 1990, 11:296.

Katzman R, et al. Develop of dementing ill. in 80 yr. old volunteer cohort. *Am Neurol* 1989, 25:317-324.

Kondo, K Yamashita I. Case study of Alz in Japan. Biol & Social advances. *Excerpta Medica* 1990, 49-53.

Shalat SL, et. al. Risk factors for Alz. disease. *Neurology* 1987, 37:1630-1633.

Soininen H, et al. Clinical and etiological aspects of senile dementia. *Eur Neurol* 1982, 21:401-410.

Korten AE, et al. Control informant agr. in case control studies of Alz. *Int. J Epidie.* 1992, 21:1121-1131.

Breteler MMB, et al. Epidemiology of Alz disease. *Epidemiol Review* 1992, 14:59-82.

Lee PN Statistics, Sutto, UK.

Reports may be obtained from the NY Academy of Medicine, 1216 Fifth Avenue, NY, NY 10020. Phone (212) 876-8200

Ref: www.forces.org/evidence/files/liars.htm

Smokers Have a Reduced Risk of Alzheimer's and Parkinson's Disease

On Forces web site (below) of the 22 studies on Alzheimer's, 15 found a reduce risk in smokers, and none found an increased risk. And smoking is clearly associated with a reduced risk of Parkinson's disease. The fact that acute administration of nicotine improves attention and information processing in AD patients adds further plausibility to the hypothesis.

Ref: \o "http://www.forces.org/evidence/files/liars.htm" http://www.forces.org/evidence/files/liars.htm

Twin Study Supports Protective Effect of Smoking for Parkinson's Disease

NEW YORK (Reuters Health) Mar 05 - Twins with Parkinson's disease (PD) who were analyzed in a new study smoked significantly less on average than did their unaffected twin sibling. This relationship was especially pronounced among monozygotic twins.

Dr. Caroline M. Tanner, of the Parkinson's Institute in Sunnyvale, California, and associates identified twins with PD using the National Academy of Sciences-National Research Council World War II Veteran Twins Registry.

Dr. Tanner' group evaluated 113 male pairs of monozygous or dizygous twins in which at least one brother had PD. Ninety-three pairs were discordant and 20 were concordant for PD.

Among discordant pairs, those without PD smoked an average of 9.7 more pack-years than the twin with PD (p = 0.026). The difference tended to be higher among the 53 monozygotic pairs than among the 60 dizygotic pairs, although the difference was not significant (p = 0.077).

Dr. Tanner's group continued to see significant differences when dose was calculated until 10 years or 20 years prior to diagnosis. They conclude that this finding refutes the suggestion that individuals who smoke more are less likely to have PD because those who develop symptoms quit smoking.

"The inverse association of smoking dose and PD can be attributed to environmental, and not genetic, causes with near certainty," the authors write.

Neurology 2002;58:581-588.

TOURETTE'S

A Cigarette Chemical Packed With Helpful Effects?

By John Schwartz
Washington Post Staff Writer
Monday, November 9, 1998; Page A03

full article can be found at:
http://stylelive.com/wp-srv/national/longterm/tobacco/stories/
nicotine110998.htm

Excerpt follows:

"Paul R. Sanberg, professor and chair of neuroscience at the University of South Florida, said about 80 percent of his patients in a study of nicotine patches for Tourette's syndrome, a neurological disorder marked by uncontrollable tics, have "shown improvement in both decreasing the frequency and the intensity of the tics" with long-term effects. In a seeming paradox, giving patients drugs that block the action of nicotine also seems to lessen their Tourette's symptoms. No one yet knows why, but it may be because nicotine desensitizes receptors it works on -- in effect making it its own blocker.

Other medical mysteries await researchers. The exceptionally high rates of smoking among people afflicted with Attention Deficit Hyperactivity Disorder (ADHD), depression and schizophrenia suggest that nicotine and similar chemicals might provide some relief. Studies have already shown an improvement in cognitive ability among schizophrenics and a greater ability to focus among ADHD patients who wear a nicotine patch.

Abbott Laboratories is working with researchers at the National Institutes of Health to study a nicotine-like drug from the skin of Amazonian frogs used for poison darts that is, in smaller doses, a highly effective painkiller. And Esther Sabban at New York University Medical College is exploring the role of nicotine in relieving the ill effects of stress on the body.

But what about addiction? Sanberg said he has given nicotine in patch form to children as young as 8 who suffer from Tourette's. "There were clearly people that didn't like the idea of giving their children nicotine and the thought that maybe they could get addicted or start smoking," he said. Nicotine in patch and gum form does not appear to carry the risk of addiction that smoking does, Sanberg said: In cigarettes, the first puff sends a potent jolt of the drug directly to the brain in about eight seconds, while patches and gum work far more slowly and consistently. "We haven't seen any addiction," Sanberg said.

Compared with the usual treatments for the disease, including potent antipsychotic drugs with side effects that can be severe, parents generally opt for the nicotine treatment, Sanberg said."

Nicotine: helping those who help themselves?

By John A. Rosecrans
Copyright 1998 Chemistry and Industry Magazine
July 6, 1998

One of the most frequently asked questions in tobacco research is 'why do people smoke?' This is a difficult question to answer. Tobacco displays the ies of an addictive substance, and it is likely that ne, the main active chemical in tobacco, plays an important role in people's addiction to smoking. The dependency induced by tobacco is curious because, despite the well-documented health risks of lung and heart disease, people consciously choose to continue smoking. Indeed, many alcoholics and cocaine and heroin addicts claim that stopping smoking was harder than breaking their other drug dependency.

A major characteristic of nicotine dependence is the behavior associated with tobacco use, especially for cigarette smokers. Smoking is often intertwined with environmental and internal cues (for example smoking after a meal, or when the telephone rings). This behavioral element makes giving up smoking even harder.

As more people have begun to question why people choose to use tobacco, it has become evident that nicotine may have beneficial effects that are 'therapeutic' rather than addictive. These more positive effects are, I believe, essential to why some people use nicotine. In other words, humans may learn that when they smoke they get something good from it, and this may explain why they continue to smoke in spite of the possible health consequences.

Addiction or self-help?

Tobacco use is similar to other drug dependencies, such as cocaine or alcohol addiction. But is nicotine really used just to get high? Research conducted by the US National Institutes of Drug Abuse has shown that nicotine administered intravenously in large doses of 13mg produced effects that were viewed as positive in some human subjects.[1] In addition, nicotine will be self-injected by rats, one of the hallmarks of a chemical that will induce dependence in humans.[2]

We have investigated smokers' abilities to detect the difference between two cigarettes with different nicotine concentrations (1.3 or 0.3mg nicotine/cigarette). [3] The subjects learned to discriminate between the cigarettes, but had difficulty explaining how they knew the differences between the cigarettes. The most distinguishing characteristic was differences in hoarseness at the back of the throat; however, the smokers were not always correct when they used this as a guide for telling one cigarette from another. On the other hand, the two different levels of nicotine caused very clear differences in the subjects' responses to a visual stimulus. [4] This indicates that the smokers were being altered neurophysiologically, but couldn't translate this effect into subjective terms.

This study gives a new view of a smoker. The subjects did not appear to be affected behaviorally, nor were they 'high'. Each smoker had difficulty explaining why they could discriminate between doses of nicotine in similar tasting cigarettes, which suggests that the nicotine was inducing a more subtle pharmacological effect.

Research in our laboratory using rats has indicated that nicotine has an unusual quality: it tends to have a 'normalizing' effect on behavior. Highly aroused rats tend to calm down, while under-aroused rats tend to be stimulated. [4] The nicotine's effects also appear to be long lasting - the rats respond differently weeks after receiving a dose of nicotine. But can the effects on rats be translated into human terms?

The average smoker inhales about 20 cigarettes a day, which averages out as about 200220 puffs/day, or about 80,000 puffs/year. Put another way, a smoker has to puff on a cigarette an average of every 4.8 min during their waking hours to maintain this behavior. It is interesting that, whether a person continues to smoke because of behavioral conditioning or the drug itself, a level of nicotine is present in the brain for most of the smoker's waking hours. Perhaps a person can learn that having a brain nicotine level is beneficial to them and may even serve a therapeutic purpose.

Pain relief

One reason why humans use tobacco may be for pain relief. Work by Mario Aceto and Billy Martin at the Virginia Commonwealth University, who showed that nicotine could act as an analgesic in mice and rats, 6 has been verified by Ovide Pomerleau and colleagues at the University of Michigan, who were among the first to suggest that nicotine acts as an analgesic in humans.[7] The way in which nicotine achieves this is not clear, although it may have some effects on the opiate system. Nicotine appears to induce analgesia by acting on internal systems that work via opiate receptors, as demonstrated by the ability of naloxone (which selectively blocks opiates) to block nicotine's effects in mice.[6] Interestingly, naloxone doesn't block nicotine's effects in rats, while mecamylamine (a compound that specifically blocks the action of nicotine) blocks the effects in both mice and rats.

More recently, the frog neurotoxin epibatidine (a chemical relative of nicotine) proved to be a significantly better pain reliever than nicotine (more than 50 times as potent).[8] Epibatidine is also blocked by both mecamylamine and naloxone, providing further evidence that these chemicals are linked to the opiate system. Abbott Laboratories has been studying a variety of nicotine analogues, one of which (ABT-594) is an extremely potent painkiller, and hopes to test these compounds in humans (see Figure 1). [9]

Anxiety and depression

Several researchers have observed that many smokers claim they smoke to relieve stress or anxiety.[10] Naomi Breslau and co-workers at the Henry Ford Hospital, Detroit, on the other hand, suggest that many smokers use tobacco to relieve an underlying depression. They evaluated levels of depression in several thousand members of a health maintenance organization and concluded that there is a powerful correlation between smoking rate and depression.[11] So, do people learn to smoke and continue to use tobacco to relieve an underlying depression or anxiety?

Research has shown that those with depression have a more difficult time stopping smoking, and that some develop depressive symptoms after nicotine tobacco use.[12] Antidepressants such as *Wellbutrin*, or, when used to treat nicotine dependence, *Zyban*, appear to help certain smokers stop using nicotine. These drugs could be substituting for nicotine's antidepressant effects in a way not dissimilar to a nicotine patch.

Other research has provided support for nicotine's role in depression. In one study, non-smoking depressed patients were given transdermal nicotine patches (17.5mg) and their sleep patterns and mood were evaluated.[13] The amount of REM (rapid eye movement), which is usually less in depression, was increased in these depressed patients. They also showed a short-term improvement in mood. Interestingly, the sleep of normal volunteers was disrupted, indicating that nicotine had a different, more positive effect in the depressed.

Other workers have suggested that the beneficial effects of nicotine may in part depend on genetic factors controlling the function of the neurotransmitter dopamine. They found a significant statistical interaction between a dopamine receptor gene (DRD4 genotype) and depression in a population of 231 smokers.[14] This work also infers that nicotine may be acting at central dopamine nerve cells, a neurotransmitter system associated with behavioral reward systems.[15] Researchers such as George Koob and co-workers at the Scripps Research Institute also point out the similarities between depression and drug dependence in general, and the fact that man may self-medicate with a variety of drugs to relieve depression. Furthermore, this research also suggests that these drugs may act on a variety of brain neurotransmitters such as serotonin and dopamine, chemicals involved in many psychiatric syndromes including depression and schizophrenia.[16]

Clearly, nicotine replacement could be beneficial in smokers who are depressed, as these studies have shown. Furthermore, there may also be a role for using the nicotine patch in depressed non-smokers.[13] However, much research needs to be conducted under a variety of conditions before the possible use of nicotine patches in depression can be implemented. Overall, these studies indicate a link between nicotine and the 'positive reward systems' such as dopamine-containing nerve cells in the brain. More importantly, as nicotine itself acts on receptors for another neurotransmitter, acetylcholine, they provide evidence for the role of these receptors in controlling behavi

Attention deficit hyperactivity disorders

Adults and adolescents with attention deficit hyperactivity disorders (ADHD) smoke more frequently than normal individuals.[17] Ed Levin and co-workers at Duke University suggested that ADHD sufferers may be using nicotine to treat their disorder. To test this hypothesis, smokers and non-smokers with ADHD were given nicotine patches (7 or 21mg/day). The researchers found a significant improvement in concentration, vigor and performance in measures of attention and timing.[17]

In a second study, these workers conducted a similar investigation on smokers and non-smokers with ADHD. They found a similar effect, which appeared to be independent of whether or not the subject was a smoker.[18] Much as with the rats described earlier, nicotine appears to be able to normalize arousal levels, so that the ADHD individual can maintain focus and attention when the brain is receiving too much information (high arousal) or possibly not enough information (low arousal).

Schizophrenia

Most counselors working in a psychiatric hospital will tell you that schizophrenics smoke an awful lot. This may be because nicotine might be acting at the brain dopamine system, one of the brain neurochemical systems that appear to be the cause of some schizophrenias (most antipsychotic drugs work by calming a hyperactive dopamine system). Another possibility is that nicotine may relieve the side effects of the drugs used to treat the disorder, or even reduce some negative effects of the schizophrenia itself. There .is some evidence to support this concept.

In addition, several psychiatrists and doctors have observed major psychotic events associated with tobacco cessation, which has been interpreted as nicotine withdrawal. Some health professionals have suggested, on the other hand, that these individuals may smoke to reduce the symptoms of behavioral disorder.

So, which came first, the behavioral disorder or chronic tobacco use? While this is difficult to answer, recent research by Robert Freedman, Sheri Leonard and co-workers at the University of Colorado has shown that schizophrenics process sensory information differently to 'normal' people.[19, 20] Unlike a schizophrenic, if a non-schizophrenic is startled by an auditory or visual stimulus, they quickly become accustomed to it if it is repeated. Research has found that when schizophrenics are given nicotine, via a patch or gum, they can cope with auditory or visual stimuli in much the same way as 'normal' people. This supports the theory that nicotine is acting in a therapeutic manner via receptors associated with the sensory habituation.

In addition, schizophrenics have fewer nicotine receptors in their brains than normal people,[21] and the expression of one of the nicotine receptor subunits (the alpha-7 unit) is also reduced in these subjects. These studies may have provided us with some important clues about the central workings of schizophrenia. First, the findings indicate that a nicotinic receptor may be at fault in at least one aspect of this behavioral syndrome - the inability of the schizophrenic to process certain kinds of sensory information. Second, the work also indicates that there may be a genetic link involving the inheritance of the alpha-7 nicotinic receptor gene from one generation to another.[19] All of this provides important clues as to why schizophrenics smoke, and may be a rationale for using nicotine (nicotine patch or gum) in non-smokers with these abnormal behavioral symptoms. Again, much careful research is needed before we can make the jump to using nicotine in the clinic.

Tourette's syndrome

Tourette's syndrome is a disorder characterized by uncontrolled speech and limb movement. Sufferers, who tend to be young adolescents, often curse and swear uncontrollably. The cause of Tourette's is still unknown, but it appears to involve problems in dopamine transmission. The syndrome is difficult to control medically, especially in patients who are resistant to drugs containing typical antipsychotic agents such as haldol or chlorpromazine.

Paul Sanberg at the University of South Florida gave a nicotine patch or gum (7mg or 2mg, respectively) to an adolescent Tourette's sufferer. The nicotine reduced the movement and speech syndrome within minutes. Interestingly, the nicotine patch attenuated the movement disorder for several days after a single application. While nicotine appears to be effective in treating Tourette's syndrome, these researchers suggest that the best use of the nicotine patch at this point is as an adjunct to antipsychotic treatment (rather than using nicotine alone), until more research is conducted.

Nicotine's success here may be a result of its unusual mode of action. When it binds to the nicotine receptors in the brain (actually members of the family of receptors sensitive to the neurotransmitter acetylcholine) it first activates them and then desensitises them, effectively turning them off (see Figure 2). [22] In addition, the ability of nicotine to activate or desensitize a receptor may also depend on the receptor's activity at the time the nicotine is administered or gets to the receptor. Thus, nicotine may tend to activate the receptor if it is inactive (as it is if there is little acetylcholine present at the receptor). On the other hand, nicotine may deactivate (desensitize) the receptor when it is very active because of a high level of acetylcholine at the receptor. Thus, nicotine may be acting to normalize the receptor in a way analogous to the observations of nicotine's action on 'high' or 'low' aroused rat behavior.

If we take this hypothesis a little further and assume that Tourette's syndrome results from an overproduction of a neurotransmitter such as dopamine, then nicotine could be acting to stabilize the dopamine nerve cell by its ability to desensitize nicotinic receptors located on it. [23] Stabilization or shutting down an overproduction of dopamine could explain why nicotine is working in this syndrome, assuming dopamine is the culprit.

More recent research by the same group, has shown that mecamylamine (which blocks the action of nicotine) is also effective in reducing Tourette's symptoms. [24] At first glance, this drug would not be expected to have this effect, as it would act at the same nicotinic receptor - in other words, the receptor would have to be activated to get the same effect. The reason mecamylamine is working, however, is the fact that it is not inducing nicotine blockade by acting at the receptor, but can block nicotine by acting directly in the channel - clogging it up (see Figure 2). Thus, mecamylamine is having the same effect as nicotine but is working at a different site. This is an important study as it provides additional support for the contention that nicotine (as well as mecamylamine) is stabilizing an overactive nerve cell which releases dopamine.

Parkinson's disease

Parkinson's disease (PD) is another condition that involves exaggerated movements, tics and rigidity. It appears to be the result of a declining dopamine nerve cell system. Once, this disease was thought to be caused by viruses, but we now realize that environmental toxicity and/or the ability of our brains to make neurotoxic substances such as 6-hydroxydopamine[25] may cause nerve cells to degenerate, reducing the amount of dopamine that can be made and released. The main treatment for this condition is the administration of the dopamine precursor l-dopa, which helps the brain synthesize more dopamine.

The role of nicotine in PD has evolved over the past 20 years. Early reports indicated that smokers were less likely to develop the disease.[26] While some work suggested that this relationship was due to differences that might arise from factors such as selective mortality rather than any specific effect of tobacco or nicotine,[27] other research evaluated much of the evidence further and concluded that the effect is real - nicotine did reduce the onset of PD.[28]

Following the initial suggestion that nicotine might be protective in the development of PD, workers such as Karl Fagerstrom at Pharmacia Research Laboratories in Helsingborg, one of the developers of nicotine gum, observed that the symptoms of PD were relieved by the administration of nicotine gum or patch.[29] This work has been repeated in other laboratories[30] with the suggestion that nicotine may somehow be acting on dopamine nerve cells destroyed by PD.[31] In other words, nicotine is most likely either increasing the central availability of dopamine or preventing the loss of neuronal dopamine at brain area sites important for movement.

However, this concept may have been partially compromised by data suggesting that there may be other chemical(s) in tobacco smoke that also produce therapeutic benefits in PD sufferers.[32] This has become more evident as the neurotoxic mechanisms underlying PD have been uncovered. Recent work has shown that levels of the enzyme monamine oxidase B (MAO B), which has been implicated in PD, are 40% lower in smokers than in non-smokers, but this[32] and other studies[33] suggest that chemicals other than nicotine in tobacco smoke may be responsible for the lowered level of MAO B. It is now evident that MAO B may be responsible for the synthesis of the neurotoxins which may lead to PD. The relationship between smoking and PD appears to be quite complex, but work with nicotine patches and the smoking studies indicate that nicotine and/or some other chemical in tobacco smoke may provide some benefits to the PD sufferer.[34]

Several studies examining the nicotine patch as a treatment for PD have produced some positive outcomes. In addition, quite a few drug companies,[35] such as SIBA Neurosciences in LaJolla,[36] are developing nicotine analogues as PD therapeutics, and have had some success in monkeys. While nicotine does appear to help protect against PD, further investigation of the other substances in smoke that may be involved needs to be done.

Alzheimer's disease

Nicotine may also have a role to play in the severe dementia of Alzheimer's disease (AD). The number of nicotine receptors in the brain is reduced by 4060% in AD patients[37-39] (a similar effect is seen in select PD patients, [40] linking these two neurological syndromes together in relation to nicotine). Workers such as Paul Newhouse and colleagues at the University of Vermont have observed that nicotine, when administered as a patch, may have some benefit as a cognitive enhancer in AD as well.[41]

The relationship between smoking and AD is not that clear. There is some suggestion of a link between smoking and a lowered risk of AD, [41] but this relationship has not always held up. Neuroscience is just beginning to evaluate the many causes of AD from genetics to immunological mechanisms. The one thing we do know about AD is that nicotine receptors in the brain are destroyed, and these somehow play a role in cognition. Abbott Laboratories has invested much in the search for cognitive enhancers and has developed one nicotine analogue, ABT-418 (see Figure 1), which may hold some promise in this area.[35]

The drug of choice?

The reasons behind a smoking habit are clearly more complex than they seem at first sight. For example, a person may smoke in response to social and environmental cues, or in order to avoid the negative effects associated with giving up. On the other hand, the smoker may be using tobacco as self-medication to relieve some underlying behavioral and/or neurological problem.

The nicotine receptors in the brain appear to have a very important role in overall brain function. These receptors are actually made up of a variety of subunits, and the number of combinations is enormous. This variety appears to be related to the genetics of a specific individual that may then choose to use nicotine via tobacco to modulate one of these receptors, which in turn will alter behavior and sensory input.

It is interesting to note that habitual nicotine use actually increases the number of nicotine receptors in the brain, probably because of the drug's receptor desensitizing effects.[42] The increase seems to reflect an adaptive capacity (acute and chronic tolerance) in the brain, which may be related to how and why nicotine can exert some benefits in constant tobacco use.[23]

The wide spectrum of nicotine's therapeutic potential is only now being discovered and there may be other effects not yet found; for example, data is now accumulating that nicotine may have beneficial effects in ulcerative colitis.[43]

Many people, who use tobacco, including smokers, do so because of some potential therapeutic benefit they receive, such as to relieve depression, schizophrenia or pain. While this appears to be one reason why some people use tobacco, we should not forget that many people engage in this behavior for other reasons, such as boredom or just to do something that is now 'antisocial'. The future for developing nicotine as a therapeutic agent, or an adjunct to other therapies, using a safe delivery system is relatively good. One of the difficulties with a chemical such as nicotine is that it has been thought of as a 'dirty drug', or 'demon drug' like heroin, which makes people addicts. We first need to pull away from this concept of demonism and treat nicotine and its analogues like any other drug. If you were to ask a clinician whether he or she would use nicotine or heroin to help the patient, the answer would be 'give the drug'. Most clinicians are objective about the drugs they use so long as they help the patient.

Another problem with future research on nicotine concerns its potential addictive properties, and how such a compound should be marketed. Pharmaceutical houses are very sensitive to this problem and might stay away from a nicotine research program because the drugs they would find could be perceived as addictive. Nicotine is also not high on the list of priorities of things to do when research resources are at a low ebb. Problems such as AIDS in the world or cocaine in the US have much higher priorities. Thus, except for a couple of companies mentioned here, we may never establish large research programs to develop new chemicals that are nicotine-like, or further evaluate the therapeutic potential of nicotine. This is frustrating to many researchers in this area, but somehow many will continue, and we will eventually learn what nicotine's full therapeutic potential is regardless of the environment.

References

1. Henningfield, J.E., & Goldberg, S.R., Pharmacol. Biochem. Behav., 1988, 30, 221-6; Henningfield, J.E., Cohen, C., & Slade, J.D., *Br. J. Addict.*, 1991, **86**, 565-9

2. Rose, J.E., & Corrigal, W.A., *Psychopharmacology*, 1997, **130**, 28-40

3. Kallman, N.M., Kaliman, M.J., Harry, G.J., Woodson, P.P., & Rosecrans, J.A., in 'Drug discrimination application in CNS pharmacology', (Eds F.C. Colpaert & J.L. Slangen), *Amsterdam: Elsevier Biomedical Press*, 1982, 211-18

4. Woodson, P.P., *et al, Pharmacol. Biochem. Behav.*, 1982, **17**, 915-20

5. Rosecrans, J.A., *Behav. Genet.*, 1995, **25**, 187-96

6. Tripathi, H.L., Martin, B.R., & Aceto, M.D., *J. Pharmacol. Exp. Therap.*, 1982, **221**, 91-6

7. Pomerleau, O.F., Turk, D.C., & Fertig, J.B., *Addict. Behav.*, 1984, **9**, 265-71

8. Bado, B., & Daly, J.W., *Mol. Pharmacol.*, 1994, **45**, 563-70

9. Bannon, A.W., *et al, Science*, 1998, **279**, 77-81

10. Kassel, J.D., & Shiffman, S., *Health Psychol.*, 1997, **16**, 359-68

11. Bressau, N., Peeterson, E.L., Schultz, L.R., Chilcoat, H.D., & Andreski, P., *Arch. Gen. Psychiat.*, 1998, **559**, 161-6

12. Glassman, A.H., *et al, JAMA*, 1990, **264**, 1546-9

13. Slin-Pascual, R.J., de la Fuente, J.R., Galicia-Polo, L., & Drucker-Colin, R., *Psychopharmacology*, 1995, **121**, 476-9

14. Lerman, C., *et al, Health Psychol.*, 1998, **17**, 56-62

15. Rosecrans, J.A., *Chem. Ind.*, 1994, 221-4

16. Markou, A., Kosten, T.T., & Koob, G.F., *Neuropsychopharmacol.*, 1998, **18**, 135-74

17. Conners, C.K., *et al, Psychopharmacol. Bull.*, 1996, **32**, 67-73

18. Levin, E.D., *et al, Psychopharmacology*, 1996, **123**, 55-63

19. Freedman, R., *et al*, *Proc. Natl Acad. Sci. USA*, 1997, **94**, 587-92

20. Leonard, S., *et al*, *Schizophr. Bull.*, 1996, **22**, 431-45

21. Freedman, B., Hall, M., Adler, L.E., & Leonard, S., *Biol. Psychiat.*, 1995, **38**, 22-33

22. Marks, M.J., Busch, J.B., & Collins, A.C., *J. Pharmacol. Exp. Therap.*, 1983, **226**, 554-64

23. Rosecrans, J.A., & Karan, L., *J. Subst. Abuse Res.*, 1992, **10**, 161-70

24. Shytle, R.D., Silver, A.A., & Sanberg, P.R., Poster presented at the International Behavioural Neuroscience Society Annual Meeting, 11-14 June 1998, Richmond, VA, US

25. Jellinger, K., Linert, L., Kienzl, E., Herlinger, E., & Youdim, M.B.H., *J. Neural. Transm.*, 1995, **46**(Suppl), 297-314

26. Baron, J.A., Neurology, 1986, **36**, 1490-6

27. Haack, D.G., Baumann, R.J., McKean, H.E., Jameson, H.D., & Turbek, J.A., *Am. J. Epidemiol.*, 1981, **114**, 191-200

28. Morens, D.M., et al, ibid, 1996, 144, 400-4

29. Fagerstrom, K.O., Pomerleau, O., Giordani, B., & Stelson, F., *Psychopharmacology*, 1994, **116**, 117-19

30. Clemens, P., Baron, J.A., Coffey, D., & Reeves, A., *ibid*, 1995, **117**, 253- 6

31. Kirch, D.G., Alho, A.M., & Wyatt, R.J., *Cell. Mol. Neurobiol.*, 1988, **8**, 285-91

32. Fowler, J.S., *et al*, *Nature*, 1996, 379, 733-6

33. Mendez-Alvarez, E., Soto-Otero, R., Sanchez-Sellero, I., & Lopez-Rivadulla Lomas, M., *Life Sci.*, 1997, 60, 1719-927

34. Shytle, R.D., Borlongan, C.V., Cahill, D.W., & Sanberg, P.R., *Med. Chem. Res.*, 1996, **6**, 555-61

35. Brioni, J.D., Decker, M.W., Sullivan, J.P., & Arneric, S.P., *Advan. Pharmacol.*, 1997, **37**, 153-214

36. Menzaghi, F., Whelan, K.T., Risbrough, V.B., Rao, T.S., & Lloyd, G.K., *J. Pharmacol. Exp. Therap.*, 1997, **280**, 393-401

37. Flynn, D.D., & Mash, D.C., *J. Neurochem.*, 1986, **47**, 1984-54

38. Nordberg, A., *et al*, *J. Neural Transm.*, 1990, **2**, 215-24

39. Whitehouse, P.J., *et al*, *Arch. Neurol.*, 1988, **45**, 722-4

40. Perry, E.K., *et al*, *J. Neurol. Neurosurg. Psychiat.*, 1987, **50**, 806-9

41. Newhouse, P.A., Potter, A., & Levin, E.D., *Drugs Aging*, 1997, **11**, 206-28

42. Balfour, D.J., & Fagerstrom, K.O., *Pharmacol. Therap.*, 1996, **72**, 51-81

43. Kennedy, L.D., *Ann. Pharmacotherap.*, 1996, **30**, 1022-3

Dr Rosecrans is Professor of Pharmacology and Toxicology and Rehabilitation Counseling, Virginia Commonwealth University, Richmond, Virginia 23298, US.

News Anchor Reports on USF Study

Below is a report on a remarkable study done at the University of South Florida by news anchor Julie Francavilla from Channel 5 in Seattle, Washington.

"Researchers from the University of South Florida found nicotine patches boost the effectiveness of drugs given to relieve the tics, verbal outbursts and hyperactivity of children afflicted with Tourette's syndrome.

They followed patients ranging in age from nine to 15 who responded poorly to haloperidol (Haldol) or other drugs commonly given to treat Tourette's. When the drug was combined with a low dose nicotine patch, the benefits of the medication increased an average of 45 percent. Patients wore the patch for 24 hours, and then removed it. Relief from symptoms occurred within three hours of administering the patch and was maintained up to 10 days after the patch was removed.

It is still unclear why nicotine reduces the involuntary movements of Tourette's, but researchers suspect it may somehow turn off the activity of a specific brain receptor that may be involved in the brain chemistry of people with Tourette's. In many cases, nicotine and medications for Tourette's can gradually be decreased or stopped by the time a patient reaches age 20. Studies showed the patch was effective in controlling symptoms 80 percent of the time.

The nicotine is delivered to the patient through a patch. This allows it to be absorbed into the blood in a way that is different than if taken by smoking or by chewing gum. The levels in the blood rise gradually and reach the maximum level in about three hours. It then gradually decreases over 24 hours. The patch used in the study contains seven milligrams of nicotine, similar to the nicotine patches available in the story."

For more information, contact:
Archie A. Silver, M.D.
USF Physicians Group
3515 E. Fletcher Ave. MDC 14
Tampa, FL 33613
(813) 974-1516

Nicotine for the treatment of Tourette's syndrome

Sanberg PR, Silver AA, Shytle RD, Philipp MK,
Cahill DW, Fogelson HM, McConville BJ.

Department of Surgery, University of South Florida College of
Medicine, Tampa 33612-4799, USA.

Recent evidence has demonstrated that nicotine may obtund the symptoms of Tourette's syndrome (TS). TS is a neuropsychiatric disorder characterized by motor and vocal tics, obsessions and compulsions, and frequently with impulsivity, distractibility, and visual-motor deficits. While neuroleptics, such as haloperidol, are most effective for treatment of the motor and vocal tics of TS, these medications have many side effects. In this article, we review the evidence, consistent with findings in animals, that administration of nicotine (either 2 mg nicotine gum or 7 mg transdermal nicotine patch) potentiates the therapeutic properties of neuroleptics in treating TS patients and that a single patch may be effective for a variable number of days. These findings suggest that transdermal nicotine could serve as an effective adjunct to neuroleptic therapy for TS.

Smoking and Schizophrenia

by Norman Swan

There's more and more interest around the world in why people with mental illness have very high rates of smoking. Is it because of stress, or could it be that tobacco is actually helping the condition? If so, it's a double-edged sword.

One example is a study of quitting cigarettes in smokers with and without schizophrenia. The researchers monitored thinking ability.

In the people who had schizophrenia, quitting was especially difficult and often didn't last long, and in addition it made their thinking ability worse — whereas in healthy individuals, thinking ability improved.

This is important for a couple of reasons. Work in Western Australia has shown that people with schizophrenia have significantly shorter lifespans than the rest of us, and one reason is their high rate of smoking-related illnesses — up to 90 per cent of these people smoke.

The second reason is that smoking may be a form of self-medication, and nicotine possibly could be used to treat people with schizophrenia. Patches have been tried and they've been disappointing, but it could point to the way to new, innovative medications based on the smoking idea.

For reference:
George TP et al ublications/store/5/0/5/7/7/8/"
Neuropsychopharmacology 2002 vol 26 pp 75-85
George TP et al American Journal of Psychiatry 2000 vol 157 pp 1835-1842

For more information:
/8.30/helthrpt/stories/s614060.htm" Health Report 22/7/2002 – Schizophrenia and smoking All in the Mind 17/3/2002 – Can smoking too much marijuana cause psychosis?

WOMEN, CHILDREN & TOBACCO

Is Smoking Bad for Eclampsia Patients?

Urinary Continine Concentration Confirms the reduced Risk of Preeclampsia with Tobacco Exposure

Preeclampsia is primarily a disease of the last trimester of pregnancy. In the mother, it is characterized by high blood pressure and proteinuria, and in severe cases headaches, blurring of vision and seizures. End-organ damage, especially to the kidneys and liver, may result if the condition is not recognized early enough, and the condition can be life threatening. Consequences for the late term fetus include diminished placental blood flow, and subsequent wasting and asymmetrical growth of the fetus. Previously known as 'toxemia' or 'toxemia of pregnancy', preeclampsia is currently also referred to as Pregnancy-Induced Hypertension, or PIH. At present, the «best» [?} cure for this disease is delivery of the preterm baby followed by intensive neonatal care for baby and intensive surgical care for the mother. [Or she could simply SMOKE, and reduce the risk by 2/3!]

Objective: We assessed tobacco exposure in nulliparous women with preeclampsia compared with that in control subjects by measuring urinary cotinine to confirm the reduced risk of preeclampsia associated with tobacco exposure during pregnancy.

Conclusion: These findings, obtained by using laboratory assay [urine continine levels], confirm the reduced risk of developing preeclampsia with tobacco exposure. (**Am J Obstet Gynecol 1999;181**:1192-6.)

Volume 34 Number 20
June 13, 2002

University Times

VOLUME 34 NUMBER 20 Copyright (c) , **University of Pittsburgh**

Physiological changes during pregnancy, preeclampsia studied

Every six minutes, a woman dies of a pregnancy complication called preeclampsia, according to the Preeclampsia Foundation. Worldwide, the disorder, which is linked to hypertension, leads to an estimated 76,000 deaths — 30,000 in Africa alone.

Women who have experienced the condition, also known as toxemia, have an even greater chance of developing the disorder in subsequent pregnancies.

The results of several clinical and basic science research studies of preeclampsia were presented by Magee-Womens Research Institute faculty at the 13th World Congress of the International Society for the Study of Hypertension in Pregnancy, which was held here recently.

Highlights of the findings include:

Condition leads to increased levels of sialic acid in blood Blood concentrations of a metabolic sugar called sialic acid are increased in women who develop preeclampsia with preterm delivery but not term delivery, Carl A. Hubel, assistant professor of obstetrics, gynecology and reproductive sciences at Pitt's School of Medicine, and his colleagues found. Preeclampsia that takes place in preterm is generally more severe than that which develops later, and is more likely to be associated with fetal growth restriction. Elevated levels of sialic acid indicate inflammation and are associated with an increased risk of atherosclerosis.

Blood samples were studied from pregnant women who had experienced preeclampsia in a previous pregnancy. Women were randomized into two groups, receiving either 60 milligrams of aspirin, an anti-inflammatory drug, or a placebo daily. Early results also indicate that the low-dose aspirin may lessen this inflammatory response.

Preeclampsia heightens risk for high blood pressure Women who have had preeclampsia appear to be at greater risk for high blood pressure and cardiovascular disease later in life, Roberta Ness, associate professor of epidemiology and obstetrics, gynecology and reproductive sciences, graduate student Patricia Agatisa and their colleagues found.

By studying heart rate, blood pressure and forearm blood flow in pregnant women who had a prior preeclampsia, women with normal pregnancies, and never-pregnant women when under stress, investigators found that having had a normal pregnancy was associated with a positive long-term effect on blood vessel behavior that was not present in women who had previous preeclamptic pregnancies or those who had never been pregnant.

Smoking found to decrease risk of preeclampsia While smoking during pregnancy has many adverse health effects on mother and fetus, it appears to decrease the risk of preeclampsia, Kristine Yoder Lain, assistant professor of obstetrics, gynecology and reproductive sciences at the School of Medicine, and her colleagues found.

Uric acid concentrations in the blood were compared among women with normal pregnancies, including smokers, nonsmokers and smokers who had quit smoking during pregnancy. Elevated levels of uric acid are observed during normal pregnancy among smokers. Higher uric acid levels also are observed in preeclampsia. Uric acid concentrations increased for all pregnant women, but the rate of increase was greatest among those who had quit smoking at the onset of pregnancy.

Other blood studies of pregnant smokers found that certain cellular components associated with blood-vessel activation called fibronectin, vascular cellular adhesion molecule-1 and intracellular adhesion molecule-1 were either reduced or increased. Reasons for a decreased risk of preeclampsia among smokers remain elusive, researchers said.

Junk Science Presses The Attack!

RESULTS: Twenty-four studies on nicotine (tobacco smoking), nine on alcohol, one on caffeine, and five on psychosocial stress were identified. All were published between 1973 and 2002., Contradictory findings were reported in the alcohol studies, and no conclusion could be reached on the basis of the caffeine study. Results from studies on psychological stress during pregnancy were inconsistent but indicated a possible modest contribution to ADHD symptoms in the offspring. **CONCLUSIONS:** Other maternal lifestyle factors during pregnancy may also be associated with these disorders. Further studies are needed to reach conclusions.

June 10 - **How Many Researchers Does It Take To Crank Out A Study That Reaches No Conclusion?** - No snappy punch line to this query but those with a mordant wit may get a chuckle out of reading the summary of this non-study. The objective was to determine whether tobacco, alcohol, caffeine or something called "psychosocial stress" during pregnancy leads to Attention Deficit Hyperactivity Disorder. Since ADHD is a disorder made up and promoted to sell dangerous psychoactive drugs to distracted parents of rambunctious boys it's not surprising that the conclusions to this effort are ephemeral. The researchers poured through 36 studies cranked out over a period of 29 years. Most, not surprisingly, dealt with maternal smoking while a handful dealt with drinking while pregnant. One examined mothers on caffeine while five looked at psychosocial stress. The provisos rain down fast and thick:

"In spite of inconsistencies..."
"Contradictory findings..."
"were inconsistent but indicated a possible..."
"methodological shortcomings..."

Out of this riot of fudge words come conclusions that actually are no conclusions at all. Tobacco smoke smoke in utero "is suspected to be associated" with ADHD while other maternal lifestyle factors "may be also associated." There is only one definitive, unequivocal statement and that occurs at the end:

Further studies are needed to reach conclusions

For this eleven researchers with silver-plated credentials were needed? Guess so, when the real purpose is to extract money from foundations and the taxpayers. For a more useful understanding of mothers and ADHD, a simple picture is worth a thousand buzz words and several hundred thousand dollars of research grants:

Am J Psychiatry 160:1028-1040, June 2003© 2003 American Psychiatric Association Reviews and Overviews **Maternal Lifestyle Factors in Pregnancy Risk of Attention Deficit Hyperactivity Disorder and Associated Behaviors: Review of the Current Evidence Karen Markussen Linnet, M.D., Søren Dalsgaard, M.D., Ph.D., Carsten Obel, M.D., Kirsten Wisborg, M.D., D.M.Sc., Tine Brink Henriksen, M.D., Ph.D., Alina Rodriguez, Ph.D., Arto Kotimaa, B.M., Irma Moilanen, M.D., Ph.D., Per Hove Thomsen, M.D., D.M.Sc., Jørn Olsen, M.D., Ph.D., and Marjo-Riitta Jarvelin, M.D., Ph.D. OBJECTIVE:** The purpose of this review was to examine the literature assessing the relationship between prenatal exposure to nicotine, alcohol, caffeine, and psycho-social stress during pregnancy to the risk of developing behavioral problems related to attention deficit hyperactivity disorder (ADHD) in childhood. **METHOD:** PubMed, MEDLINE, EMBASE, and PsycINFO were searched systematically. Studies using DSM diagnostic criteria and other validated diagnostic or screening instruments for ADHD and those examining ADHD symptoms were included. A narrative approach was used because the studies differed too much in methods and data sources to permit a quantitative meta-analysis. **RESULTS:** Twenty-four studies on nicotine (tobacco smoking), nine on alcohol, one on caffeine, and five on psychosocial stress were identified. All were published between 1973 and 2002. In spite of inconsistencies, the studies on nicotine "indicated" a greater risk of ADHD-related disorders among children whose mothers smoked during pregnancy. Contradictory findings were reported in the alcohol studies, and no conclusion could be reached on the basis of the caffeine study. Results from studies on psychological stress during pregnancy were inconsistent but indicated a possible modest contribution to ADHD symptoms in the offspring. Many studies suffered from methodological shortcomings, such as recall bias, crude or inaccurate exposure assessments, low statistical power, and lack of or insufficient control of confounders. A general lack of information on familial psychopathology also limited the interpretations. **CONCLUSIONS:** Exposure to tobacco smoke in utero is suspected to be associated with ADHD and ADHD symptoms in children. Other maternal lifestyle factors during pregnancy may also be associated with these disorders. Further studies are needed to reach conclusions.

Maternal Smoking, Body Mass Index and Neural Tube Defects

K Kallen
Tornblad Institute, University of Lund, Sweden.

The Swedish health registries were used to investigate a possible effect on the incidence of neural tube defects (NTDs) of maternal smoking and maternal body mass index (BMI) (kg/m2). Among 1,199,701 infants born in 1983-1993 with known smoking exposure in early pregnancy, 621 infants with NTDs

298 / THE HEALTH BENEFITS OF TOBACCO

were selected. After controlling for year of birth, maternal age, parity, education level, BMI, and immigrant status (yes/no), **a highly significant, protective effect of maternal smoking on the incidence of NTDs was found.** The adjusted odds ratios (OR) and (95% confidence intervals (CI)) for maternal smoking among infants with NTDs (total), anencephaly, and spina bifida were 0.75 (0.61-0.91), 0.49 (0.28-0.85), and 0.76 (0.61-0.95), respectively. A protective dose-response effect of smoking was indicated but was not statistically significant. The association between NTDs and maternal BMI found in earlier studies was supported. Women with BMI >26.0 were found to be at higher risk of having an infant with NTD compared with women in other BMI classes (adjusted OR=1.35, 95% CI 1.00-1.83). For women with BMI >or =29, the corresponding odds ratio was 1.29 (0.81- 2.05). No obvious explanation was found, either for the detected association between NTDs and BMI, or for the protective effect of maternal smoking.

California Tobacco Trashers

SCIENTIFIC FRAUD

IN THE CALIFORNIA EPA REPORT
"HEALTH EFFECTS OF EXPOSURE TO ENVIRONMENTAL TOBACCO SMOKE"

PART 1: CHAPTERS 3, 4, AND 5:

DEVELOPMENTAL TOXICITY AND REPRODUCTIVE EFFECTS

We now have direct and incontrovertible proof of deliberate scientific misconduct and concealment of crucial evidence exonerating smoking by the anti-smoking health establishment,

In May of this year, I sent in public comments on the California EPA ETS report. The authors of Chapters 3 (Gayle Windham and Mari Golub), 4 (Kirsten Waller), and 5 (Gayle Windham and Mari Golub) completely glossed over my criticisms. I sent them a copy of my article, "How the anti-smokers lie about smoking and pregnancy," as well as my comments on their report.

In particular, they ignored the solid epidemiological evidence that the purported poor perinatal outcome in smokers is entirely attributable to a fatal methodological defect of the anti-smokers' own studies, namely their failure to detect chorioamnionitis because they failed to perform placental pathological examinations. NONE OF THE ANTI-SMOKERS' STUDIES HAVE BEEN DONE CORRECTLY, BECAUSE OF THIS DEFICIENCY. And, because of their epidemiological malpractice, they missed about 90% of cases, which they then proceeded to falsely blame on smoking.

Windham and Golub deliberately ignored this issue with their disingenuous response: "The document notes that at a minimum, maternal age, prior history of pregnancy loss, and socioeconomic status should be considered as potential confounders." My major point is that it has been demonstrated that these are insufficient.

And, "The relative contribution of these other confounders has not been established, but their distribution by ETS exposure status must vary in order them to confound the association. It is not clear why this would be so with these particular factors."

The relative contribution of chorioamnionitis HAS been established by the work of RL Naeye, and the anti-smokers have systematically concealed it.

Naeye: "We recently found no significant association between maternal smoking and either stillbirths or neonatal deaths when information about the underlying disorders, obtained from placental examinations, was incorporated into the analysis. Similar analyses found no correlation between maternal smoking and pre term birth. The most frequent initiating causes of stillbirth, and neonatal death are acute chorioamnionitis, disorders that produce chronic low blood flow from the uterus to the placenta, and major congenital malformations. There is no credible evidence that cigarette smoking has a role in the genesis of any of these disorders." Naeye's study population is the 56,000+ pregnancies of the Collaborative Perinatal Study. (RL Naeye. Disorders of the placenta, fetus, and neonate, diagnosis and clinical significance. New York: CV Mosby Co., 1992).

And, it IS clear why the rates of chorioamnionitis would vary by ETS status: because those most exposed to passive smoke are those who are the most like smokers themselves: "Acute chorioamnionitis is the largest contributor to the poor pregnancy outcomes of black women and women who have low socioeconomic status," and it is "the most common cause of prettier labor wherever it has been studied," in the words of Naeye. (Acute chorioamnionitis and the disorders that produce placental insufficiency. In: Monographs in Pathology No., Pathology of Reproductive Failure. FT Kraus et al, eds. Williams and Wilkins 1991. Ch 10, pp 286-307).

The anti-smokers' scientific fraud is long-standing and systematic. NONE of the anti-smokers' studies or reviews address the role of chorioamnionitis. For example, it is entirely absent from the widely cited review by DiFranza (Effect of maternal cigarette smoking on pregnancy complications and Sudden Infant Death Syndrome. J Fam Pract 1995 Apr;40(4):385-394). Incidentally, DiFranza was on the witness list for the Full Committee hearing on Tobacco Restrictions and Youth, Sep 16, 1997, by Sen. John McCain. And, DiFranza ought to be interrogated about why his supposedly exhaustive research of the literature failed to turn up any work by Naeye dating after 1976.

In fact, the anti-smokers have conducted defective studies for nearly 40 years, ignoring the early work by WA Blanc which demonstrated the necessity of placental examinations (Amniotic infection syndrome. Pathogenesis, morphology, and significance in circumnatal mortality. Clin Obstet Gynecol 1959;2:705).

Windham and Golub have committed an additional element of fraud by falsely attributing perinatal illness and death to simple "low birth weight," which are actually healthy births.

Their central premise that "if the distribution of birthright is shifted lower with ETS exposure, as it appears to be with active smoking, infants who are already compromised may be pushed into even higher risk categories. Low birthright is associated with many well recognized problems for infants, and is strongly associated with perinatal mortality," is bogus.

Low birth weight in the absence of chorioamnionitis or other actual disease, is of negligible clinical significance. THE KEY FACTOR IS THE PRESENCE OR ABSENCE OF DISEASE, specifically of chorioamnionitis, and statistical sleights of hand purporting to predict illness by shifting the means of bell curves are pure deceit.

It is the purpose of REAL science to distinguish false and artifactual associations from genuine ones, but Windham and Golub, along with their fellow anti-smokers, have deliberately obscured and confounded these distinctions, in order to make malicious and unfounded accusations against smoking. And, the authors refused to acknowledge the evidence or address the points when these were directly presented to them, as well as continuing the ongoing conspiracy of silence about RL Naeye's work.

Elsewhere, Windham and Golub made no mention of the correction I sent in to change the words "vitamin E" to "folic acid." Nor did they mention my summary of studies of active smoking and neural tube defects, which, even in the absence of controlling for folic acid in any of them, showed no relation between active smoking and neural tube defects.

And, in other responses, Windham and Golub simply brushed off my criticisms that the existing evidence was deficient.

For example, Helicobacter pylori infection in children, besides reducing adult height by slowing the growth spurt, could well affect fetal growth as well. But studies of this have not been done, and should be, before any conclusions are drawn. Windham and Golub merely offered an evasive, non-scientific argument from intimidation that "The evidence for an effect of maternal smoking is not detailed in this document, but it has been clearly shown in numerous studies and is accepted by medical experts." Those studies are not reputable when they leave out important factors, and the so-called "experts" embrace them out of nothing but malice.

Physical activity and violence during pregnancy are issues which should be addressed in particular for spontaneous abortion. Again, such studies have not been performed, and should be, before any conclusions are drawn.

Windham and Golub just blew them off under the same evasive response they gave for perinatal mortality: "The document notes that at a minimum, maternal age, prior history of pregnancy loss, and socioeconomic status should be considered as potential confounders. The relative contribution of these other confounders has not been established, but their distribution by ETS exposure status must vary in order them to confound the association." [Meaning, `what we don't know we don't care about, because we want to find smoking guilty.'] It is not clear why this would be so with these particular factors" [when socioeconomic confounding is a clear probability].

In Chapter 4, Kirsten Waller ignored my criticism that SIDS, by definition, is not a disease; it is merely a catchall for any unknown cause of death. As such, it is extremely vulnerable to confounding by uninvestigated socioeconomic factors. Like Windham and Golub, she clearly views it as acceptable to recklessly exploit confounding factors, in flagrant disregard for the requirements of good science.

Waller also refused to address the issue that Helicobacter pylori infection in children reduces adult height by slowing the growth spurt; and that more studies should therefore be done.

And, in Chapter 5, Windham and Golub summarized my objection that this report ignored its own statement that "covariates related to sexual practices are important to consider, including frequency of coitus,..." by relying on defective studies that did not consider those covariates to falsely suggest that passive smoking reduces fertility in women. And then, just as they did in their report, they simply ignored it!

They deliberately concealed the evidence I submitted from RL Naeye's study, which unlike their studies DID consider frequency of coitus, and which consequently exonerated active smoking. "However, this association completely disappeared when confounding risk factors were taken into consideration. The two confounding risk factors that were responsible for the delay that smokers experienced in becoming pregnant were being over 34 years in age and having blue-collar employment outside of the home."

Maternal Smoking References

Seidman DS, Ever-Hadani P, Gale R **Effects of maternal smoking and age on congenital anomalies.** Obstet Gynecol Dec. 1990;76:1046-1050. Israel, 1921 major defects, smokers 0.94 (0.62-1.43); minor 1,06 (0.90-1.25).

Kelsey JL, Dwyler T, Halford TR, Bracken MB **Maternal smoking and congenital malformations: An epidemiological study.** J Epidemiol Commun Health 1978:32:102-107. Retrospective case-control, random control at "several hospital in Connecticut," 1369 cases. 1-10 cigarettes 1.0, 11-20 1.1, 21-30c 1.4, >/= 31c 1.9; all smokers 1.10 (0.97-1.26).

Evans DR, Newcombe RG, Campbell H. **Maternal smoking habits and congenital malformations: a population study.** BMJ 1979 Jul 21;2:171-173. Cardiff,

Wales Noted association with low class. Rates for all 1864 cases: 0 cigarettes 2.8%, 1-9 2.5%, 10-19 2.8%, >/= 20 3.0% [calculated relative risk for smokers 0.89, 1.0, 1.07].

MacDonald AD, Armstrong BG, Sloan M. **Cigarette, alcohol, and coffee consumption and congenital defects.** AJPH Jan 1992;82(1) : 91-93. 1928 total. 1-9 cigarettes 1.14 (1.0-1.4), 10-19 1.08 (0.9-1.2), 20+ 1.02 (0.9-1.2).

Christianson RE. **The relationship between maternal smoking and the incidence of congenital anomalies.** Am. J of Epidemiol 1980;112(5):684-695. Kaiser Foundation. *"There was no significant differences in the incidence of congenital anomalies" overall.* 2077 total cases. RRs white light smokers, male child 1.03, female 0.91; heavy smoker m 1.22, f 1.05; black ls m 0.92, f 0.95; hs m 1.18, f 1.11.

Heinonen OP, Slone D, Shapiro S, eds. **Birth defects and drugs in pregnancy.** Littleton, MA: Publishing Sciences Group, 1977. Collaborative Perinatal Project prospective. 2277 cases. All malformations, 1050 white 14 cigarettes 0.9, 15-29 1.0, >/= 30 0.9; 1097 black 1.0 1.0 1.0.

Van Den Eeden SK, Karagas MR, Daling JR, Vaughan TL. **A case-control study of maternal smoking and congenital malformations.** Paediatr Perinatal Epidemiol 1990;4:147- 155. 3048 malformations, smokers 1.0 (0.9-1.1).

Shiono, PH, Klebanoff MA, Berendes HW. **Congenital malformations and maternal smoking during pregnancy.** Teratol 1986;34:65-71. Kaiser-Premanente prospective. 5624 total cases: 592 major, smokers 1.0 (0.8-1.2); 4032 minor, smokers 0.9 (0.8-0.9).

Malloy MH, Kleinman JC, Blakewell JM, Schramm WF, Land GH. **Maternal smoking during pregnancy: No association with congenital malformations in Missouri.** AJPH 1989 Sep:79 (9):1243-1246. Total 10,223, smokers 0.98 (0.94-1.03).

LESS THAN 1,000 CASES, NOT SHOWN ON GRAPH:

Andrews J, McGarry JM. **A community study of smoking in pregnancy.** J Obstet Gynaecol Br Commonw 1972 Dec;79 (12):1057-1073. Cardiff, Wales. 509 cases. Non-smokers 2.37%, smokers 2.73% abnormal infants.

Himmelberger DU, Brown BW, Cohen EN. **Cigarette smoking during pregnancy and the risk of spontaneous abortion and congenital anomaly.** Am J Epidemiol 1978;108 (6) : 470- 479. Trace Anesthetic Study, retrospective mail survey of health professionals, 935 cases, All smokers from 0.90 to 2.34, depending on parity and age.

Courtesy of Carol Thompson 08/23/93
Smokers' Rights Action Group
P.O. Box 259575
Madison, WI 53725-9575

CANCER

Blaming Smoking Instead of Radiation

January 30, 2002 - <u>**RADIATION FROM MEDI-CAL PROCEDURES IN THE PATHOGENESIS OF CANCER AND ISCHEMIC HEART DISEASE**</u> - Does smoking cause lung cancer? We realise that just asking the question (as opposed to making an emphatic statement) gets antismokers to go ballistic against heresy. However, we are not talking about religion, fanaticism, or junk science. According to *real* science, the question is *still open*. Here is further support for the co-factor point we made on our <u>recent position paper</u>. Dr. Gofman is a scientist with impressive credentials (that include both a PhD and an MD, important scientific discoveries, and retirement as a full professor from Berkeley) -- and no connection with Big Tobacco.

He states that ionising radiation in even low-dose medical applications is a *necessary* co-factor in the majority of cases of both cancer and ischemic heart disease. For example, he states that in 1993, radiation was a co-factor in 63% of the deaths from ischemic heart disease in males and in 78% of females. For all cancer deaths combined in 1988, he says radiation was a co-factor in 74% of male cancer deaths and 50% of all female cancer deaths.

Although he does not deny that smoking is an important co-factor in lung cancer, smoking is **not** as significant as a co-factor *as medical radiation is*. Moreover, in the absence of radiation, smoking would need to be *combined with other important co-factors* (such as genes, or diet) *to cause lung cancer*. Despite the impeccable credentials, however, Gofman has received only sporadic attention from media and medical establishment. Obviously the government, the physicians, and the big medical radiation supply corporations don't like what he has to say. People **must** believe that *smoking is the main cause of lung cancer* – and that political agenda **must** override any consideration on integrity of science, truth, and information -- let alone menial values such as liberty and choice of lifestyle.

OTHER DISEASES AND CONDITIONS

Gulf War Syndrome - Blame it on Tobacco!

THOUSANDS OF US TROOPS SENT HOME FOR UNEXPLAINED MEDICAL REASONS

According to the Washington Post, "more than 6,000 service members" have been sent back to either Germany or the US "due to medical reasons." This is very much at odds with US stated casualties of only 1,124 for the same period. About a 100 of the mysterious 4,500 soldiers with medical problems have died or become incapacitated due to toxic shock, deceptively labeled as pneumonia by US military spokesmen. A large portion of these toxic shock cases were reported to have been related to the soldiers recently taking up smoking during their stint in Iraq. Doctors in Germany have been ordered to not make comments about the toxic shock, but they know this is something much more dangerous than mere pneumonia. Is it another reaction to the vaccines given troops prior to departure, or a response to the many health threats that abound in a chemical and biological war ground? There is enough depleted uranium expended in Iraq to cause many health problems, which could be one explanation. Some of the medical casualties are mental cases as well. The conditions in Iraq are very stressing to front line troops, many of which do not have access to regular food or cool water in 120-degree weather for months at a time. They often have to buy ice from Iraqi civilians jut to get a cool drink. No wonder US field grade officers are getting a bad reputation among the troops for "not taking care of their own."

Nitric Oxide Mediates a Therapeutic Effect of Nicotine in Ulcerative Colitis

Green JT, Richardson C, Marshall RW, Rhodes J, McKirdy HC, Thomas GA, Williams GT

Department of Gastroenterology, University Hospital of Wales, Cardiff, UK; Department of Surgery, University Hospital of Wales, Cardiff, UK; Department of Pharmacology and Therapeutics, University of Wales College of Medicine, Cardiff, UK; Dep.

[Record supplied by publisher]

BACKGROUND: Ulcerative colitis is a condition of nonsmokers in which nicotine is of therapeutic benefit. AIMS: To examine the in vitro effect of nicotine on colonic smooth muscle activity and the role of nitric oxide (NO) as a mediator. METHODS: Nicotine, 1-10 &mgr;M, was administered to strips of circular muscle from the distal sigmoid colon of 9 patients with active ulcerative colitis and 18 with colorectal cancer. The effect of electrical field stimulation (EFS) was examined before nicotine was added. Finally L-NAME, a NO synthetase inhibitor, was added before nicotine was administered again. RESULTS: Muscle strips developed similar spontaneous resting tone. In response to EFS, ulcerative colitis tissue developed lower tensions than the controls. Nicotine significantly reduced the resting tone and peak tension after EFS, with a greater effect in controls. With L-NAME, peak tensions were increased more in ulcerative colitis than controls, and nicotine produced a much smaller reduction. CONCLUSIONS: Nicotine reduces circular muscle activity, predominantly through the release of nitric oxide-this appears to be 'up-regulated' in active ulcerative colitis. These findings may explain some of the therapeutic benefit from nicotine (and smoking) in ulcerative colitis and may account for the colonic motor dysfunction in active disease.

Ulcerative Colitis is Associated with Non-Smoking

There is no disease known to man that the smokophobics do not try to link with smoking. Two of their targets are ulcerative colitis and Crohn's disease. Using weak studies, they proclaimed that there was indeed a "relationship" between both Crohn's and ulcerative colitis. But in a dual meta-analysis of Crohn's Disease (CD) and ulcerative colitis (UC), former smokers had no less risk for CD than current smokers, while their risk increased greatly for UC. This would indicate the possibility (although it cannot be proved) that they had been protected from ulcerative colitis by smoking.

About 90% of the victims of ulcerative colitis are non-smokers. They are at 3.5 times greater risk than smokers to contract the disease. These are not just idle statistics as there is a clear relationship between this disease and colorectal cancer later in life. But it gets even grimmer. Women and men with UC have respectively a 9.5 and <u>45.5</u> times greater risk of liver and gallbladder cancer, and 31 times the risk of primary sclerosing cholangitis (inflammation of the gall bladder). These diseases have a grim prognosis. Overall cancer risk for these bowel conditions is 1.8 times that of the general population, which is, while barely significant, <u>more than the alleged excess risk of cancer to smokers</u>.

For reasons unknown, ulcerative colitis rates are five times higher among non-smoking Mormons than in the general population. With the above statistics, it would appear, but again it cannot be proved, that if the anti-smokers get their way and practically everyone is forced to quit, there will be an <u>increase</u> in ulcerative colitis and consequently an increase in bowel cancer – at least for Mormons and probably the rest of us.

Carol Thompson of the *Smokers' Rights Action Group* has uncovered some interesting statistics concerning ulcerative colitis and <u>the danger of quitting smoking</u>. In fact, a recent review of 56 studies from 1930 to 1990 has shown that, while the ratio of male to female cases has remained the same in children, in adults <u>UC has changed from mainly female to a male preponderance</u>. What could cause such a strange flip in susceptibility to a disease? Before answering the question, is there any evidence of a similar reversal in any other countries or is it just in the U.S.? This curious phenomenon has also been seen in Denmark, Iceland, and Sweden. In Japan, where few women smoke, UC is still mainly a female disease.

If you can come up with a better answer than the following, please enlighten me. The anti-tobacco propaganda has been pervasive all over the world. If you travel much, and you smoke, you can't help but notice that there is little difference between the restrictive rules in Switzerland, Panama, Mexico and the U.S. It is world wide – and getting more restrictive monthly. Since there are more male than female smokers in all countries, the rate of cessation must be higher among men, or at least in absolute numbers of quitters. This, in my opinion, makes a pretty good, but not conclusive, case **for** smoking to prevent this terrible disease.

Courtesy of Carol Thompson 08/23/93
Smokers' Rights Action Group
P.O. Box 259575
Madison, WI 53725-9575

Other Publications and Articles

Calkins BM. **A meta-analysis of the role of smoking in inflammatory bowel disease.** Dig Dis Sci 1989 Dec;34(12):1841-1854.

Collins RH et al. **Colon cancer surveillance in patients with ulcerative colitis. A critical review.** NEJM 1987;316:1654-1658.

Ekbom A et al. **Ulcerative colitis and colorectal cancer.** NEJM 1990;323:1228-1233.

Garland CF et al. **Incidence rates of ulcerative colitis and Crohn's disease in fifteen areas of the United States.** Gastroenterol 1981;81:1115-1124.

Korelitz BI. **Where do we stand on drug treatment for ulcerative colitis?** Ann Internal Med 1992 Apr

15;116(8):692-694.

Nugent FW, Haggitt RC, Gilpin PA. **Cancer surveillance in ulcerative colitis.** Gastroenterol 1991;100(5):1241-1248.

Prior P et al. **Cancer morbidity in ulcerative colitis.** Gut 1982;23:490-497.

Rasmussen HH et al. **Primary sclerosing cholangitis in patients with ulcerative colitis.** Scand J Gastroenterol 1992;27:732-736.

Ritchie JK et al. **Biliary tract carcinoma associated with ulcerative colitis.** Q J Medicine 1974;170:263-279.

Rudra T et al. **Does smoking improve colitis?** Scand J Gastroenterol 1989;24 (suppl 170):61-63.

Stonnington CM et al. **Chronic ulcerative colitis: incidence and prevalence in a community.** Gut 1987;28:402-409.

Tysk C, Jrnerot G. **Has smoking changed the epidemiology of ulcerative colitis?** Scand J Gastroenterol 1992;27:508-512.

Nicotine Therapy for Memory Loss

Doctors Test Post-Bypass Memory Drugs
Mon Nov 4, 3:32 PM ET
By LAURAN NEERGAARD, AP Medical Writer

WASHINGTON (AP) - Call it brain fog, that loss of memory and thinking ability that strikes tens of thousands of patients after open-heart surgery, and sometimes other big operations, every year.

Now doctors are studying if giving patients certain drugs just before a heart bypass could prevent this mental decline by essentially protecting the patients' brain cells from the rigors of surgery.

The clinical trials mark a turning point: For decades, doctors didn't know what to make of patient complaints that in getting their hearts fixed, something hurt their brains.

Today, few doubt it's a real problem that affects not just heart patients but those undergoing other major surgeries, such as hip or knee replacements. Often, patients recover. But one study found 42 percent of heart-bypass patients suffer significant drops in mental sharpness that can last not just months but years. Other research suggests 10 percent of hip-replacement patients suffer similar mental decline.

In some ways this "postoperative cognitive dysfunction" is a byproduct of the modern operating room. As surgery — particularly the half-million heart bypasses performed every year — has become increasingly successful, aftershocks such as a muddled brain draw more concern.

"It's a big quality of life issue," says Dr. James Cottrell, president of the American Society of Anesthesiologists.

No one knows yet what's to blame. It may be that only certain people are at high risk, such as those whose brain blood vessels are starting to clog and something about surgery speeds up the disease.

For now, suspects range from the heart-lung machine that circulates bypass patients' blood — it can dislodge tiny bits of fat, blood clots or air bubbles that flow to the brain — to the inflammation and post-surgery fever that are a risk after any major operation.

Surgery's stresses spark inflammation and other reactions that "in some ways is the body's way of healing itself," explains Dr. Mark Newman, anesthesiology chairman at Duke University and a leading expert on post-surgery mental decline. "But the question is if it goes beyond a certain level, do you end up with problems?"

That's where much of the prevention research centers: If surgery even temporarily blocks oxygen in part of the brain or sparks severe inflammation, the body reacts with a chemical cascade that injures or kills brain cells.

Newman and other scientists are studying if injecting patients with one of three different medications before a bypass could block that chain reaction and spare brain cells:

—Two small studies suggest lidocaine, normally used for irregular heartbeat, can prevent bypass patients' brain fog. Duke now is testing 250 bypass patients, half given lidocaine and half not, to see who has better brain function a year after surgery. Newman says lidocaine might work by blocking a pathway that lets toxic doses of calcium flood into oxygen-deprived brain cells.

—Certain levels of magnesium seem to block that toxicity, too, as well as lessen cell damage from inflammation. So, using federal money, Duke is enrolling 400 bypass patients into a study to see if magnesium might block brain fog.

—Initial testing of an experimental drug called pexelizumab, thought to block an inflammation-causing immune system protein, showed bypass patients who received the drug had slightly less mental decline. Duke and several other hospitals are participating in a 3,000-patient study of pexelizumab, sponsored by the drug makers Alexion Pharmaceuticals and Procter & Gamble.

Some companies also are testing if filters put onto heart-lung machines can help by keeping debris from flowing to the brain.

Until those studies are done, Newman advises patients worried about coming surgery to ask their anesthesiologists about one step believed to lower brain risk — rewarming their cooled-down bodies more slowly than usual after the operation is done.

The key is intense temperature monitoring that tells when the brain, which warms faster than other organs, reaches 98.6 degrees, Newman explains. At that point, doctors should stop warming and let other organs gradually reach normal temperature on their own.

APPENDIX B

POTENTIAL GAINS IN LIFE EXPECTANCY

UNITED STATES

Small gains at national level - THE EFFECT OF A REDUCTION IN LEADING CAUSES OF DEATH: POTENTIAL GAINS IN LIFE EXPECTANCY - Tsai SP, Lee ES, Hardy RJ. - Am J Public Health. 1978 Oct;68(10):966-71.

WHEN APPLIED TO THE ENTIRE POPULATION
Reduction by 30% of cardiovascular disease: 24 months
Reduction by 30% of melanomas: 8 months, 15 days
Reduction by 30% of traffic accidents: 2 months, 15 days
... AND WHEN THE ABOVE IS APPLIED TO THE 15 to 70 YEARS AGE RANGE:
Red. by 30% of cardiovascular disease: 5 months, 7 days
Reduction by 30% of melanomas: 3 months, 6 days
Reduction by 30% of traffic accidents: 1 month, 16 days

The potential gains in total expectation of life and in the working life ages among the United States population are examined when the three leading causes of death are totally or partially eliminated. The impressive gains theoretically achieved by total elimination do not hold up under the more realistic assumption of partial elimination or reduction. The number of years gained by a new-born child, with a 30 per cent reduction in major cardiovascular diseases would be 1.98 years, for malignant neoplasms 0.71 years, and for motor vehicle accidents 0.21 years. Application of the same reduction to the working ages, 15 to 70 years, results in a gain of 0.43, 0.26, and 0.14 years, respectively for the three leading causes of death. Even with a scientific break-through in combating these causes of death, it appears that future gains in life expectancies for the working ages will not be spectacular. The implication of the results in relation to the current debate on the national health care policy is noted.

PMID: 717606 [PubMed - indexed for MEDLINE]

Minimal gain with the elimination of cancer in the United States - PERSON-YEARS OF LIFE LOST DUE TO CANCER IN THE UNITED STATES, 1970 AND 1984 - Horm JW, Sondik EJ. - Division of Cancer Prevention and Control, National Cancer Institute, Bethesda, MD 20892 - Am J Public Health. 1989 Nov;79(11):1490-3.

WHEN APPLIED TO THE ENTIRE POPULATION 8,4 DAYS

The number of deaths due to cancer in the United States reached an all-time high of 453,450 deaths in 1984 and, due to the dynamics of population growth, will continue to increase if the risk of dying from cancer does not change. Between 1970 and 1984, the total Person-Years of Life Lost (PYLL), the sum of the difference between the actual age at death and the expected remaining lifetime for each person who died of cancer, increased for most cancer sites as well as for all sites combined. In 1984, 6,881,281 person-years of life were lost due to cancer deaths, up from 5,303,668 in 1970. The exceptions are those cancers for which there has been major progress in either prevention or treatment; e.g., stomach and cervix uteri (prevention) and testicular, Hodgkin's disease, leukemia, and childhood cancers (treatment). The Average Years of Life Lost (AYLL) per person dying from cancer in 1984 was generally less than in 1970. Overall, each person who died from cancer in 1984 died 15.2 years earlier than his/her life expectancy. The greatest loss was for those who died of childhood cancers (66.9 years earlier), followed by testicular cancer (35.8 years earlier). The least loss relative to the expectation of life was for those who died of prostate cancer. The 25,400 men who died from prostate cancer in 1984 died an average of nine years earlier than otherwise expected.

PMID: 2817158 [PubMed - indexed for MEDLINE]

This is very impressive - especially from the emotional point of view -- particularly when the good old trick of mentioning children is used. Let us observe, however, how we get manipulated. The 6,881,281 years of life lost, when multiplied by the 365 days of the year (= 2,511,667,565 - which is even more impressive: over 2 and a half billion days!) dwindle to just 8.38 per person (theoretical, of course) when divided by the great US population mass, here considered at 300 million people. Moreover, let us not forget that the above-mentioned 453,450 "deaths" would have occured anyway (because people die!); those deaths would have occurred -- always theoretically and in average -- 8.4 days later!

TEXAS

POTENTIAL GAINS IN LIFE EXPECTANCIES BY PARTIAL ELIMINATION OF LEADING CAUSES OF DEATH IN TEXAS - Tsai SP, Lee ES. - Tex Rep Biol Med. 1978;36:185-96.

BETWEEN 15 AND 70 YEARS OF AGE

Elimination of 50% of cardiovascular disease: between 6 and 12 months
Elimination of 50% of cancer: 3 months
Elimination of 50% of traffic accidents: less than 3 months

Potential gains in life expectancies among Texas population by partial elimination of 3 major causes of death are examined on the basis of the available statistics from the population census and mortality statistics for 1970. Contrary to the popular anticipation of longer potential gains, the results are not particularly encouraging. The number of years of life that would be gained during the working ages by 50% elimination of major cardiovascular diseases is less than 1/2 of 1 year, about 1/4 of 1 year by 50% elimination of malignant neoplasms, and less than 1/4 of 1 year by 50% elimination of motor vehicle accidents. Even with a scientific breakthrough in combating those causes of death it appears that future gains in life expectancies for working ages will not be spectacular. The implications of the results in relation to the current debate on the national health policy are discussed.

PMID: 725791 [PubMed - indexed for MEDLINE]

FINLAND

If the days are divided by 365 and by the few (5 or 6 million) inhabitants of the country, that gains are miserable even in Finland - THE INCREASE IN WORKING YEARS DUE TO ELIMINATION OF CANCER AS A CAUSE OF DEATH - Hakulinen T, Teppo L. - Int J Cancer. 1976 Apr 15;17(4):429-35.

FOR THE ENTIRE POPULATION

TOTAL ELIMINATION OF LUNG CANCER:
8.9 HOURS

TOTAL ELIMINATION OF STOMACH CANCER:
6.2 HOURS

TOTAL ELIMINATION OF LEUKAEMIA:
6.6 HOURS

TOTAL ELIMINATION OF BREATS CANCER:
4.6 HOURS

TOTAL ELIMINATION OF ALL FORMS OF CANCER, AND OF ALL "CANCER-RELATED RISKS"
2.38 DAYS

The relative significance of various forms of cancer in terms of causing death is analysed by estimation of the increase in person-years of working age (20-64 years) following elimination of the disease. Methods based upon the theory of competing risks are applied to the statistics on causes of death in Finland during the years 1966-70. It is estimated that if there were no lung cancer (the commonest type of cancer in both morbidity and mortality statistics in males in Finland) the annual deaths saved would yield 5,900 working years (both sexes combined) [5,600 years x 365 days =2,044,000 days; 2,044,000 days : 5.5 million people = 0.371 days gained per person, that is, 8.9 hours]. Leukaemia and cancer of the stomach would be next in rank order, with figures of respectively 4,000 and 3,900 working years more. Female cancer with the highest incidence, that of the breast, would be characterized by 2,900 additional working years. The significance of types of cancer that affect young people is stressed in these calculations: leukaemia, brain tumours and lymphomas (both sexes combined) are 6th, 12th and

11th respectively in the statistics of cancer causes of death, but 2nd, 4th and 6th respectively in the list of additional working years to be gained by elimination of the disease. On the other hand, cancer of the prostate, 3rd in males according to the annual numbers of cancer deaths, would take the 15th position for the increase in working years in males. If no risk of cancer existed, the annual deaths saved would produce 36,000 working years [2.38 days for each inhabitant of Finland], a figure exceeded only by those for cardiovascular diseases (55,000 working years) and accidents (51,000 working years). The results indicate that no practical differences exist between the results derived under the assumptions of various models for competing risks, but that the exclusion of competing risks may result in considerable degrees of bias in estimation if the population has a high general mortality.

PMID: 1279036 [PubMed - indexed for MEDLINE]

CANADA

The gains for Canada? See above - PREMATURE DEATHS IN CANADA: IMPACT, TRENDS AND OPPORTUNITIES FOR PREVENTION - Wigle DT, Mao Y, Semenciw R, McCann C, Davies JW. - Laboratory Centre for Disease Control, Health and Welfare Canada, Ottawa, Ontario - Can J Public Health. 1990 Sep-Oct;81(5):376-81.
THE ENTIRE POPULATION
TOTAL ELIMINATION OF:
Coronary diseases, traffic accidents, violence, cardiovascular disease, lung cancer, perinatal conditions, as well as control of tobacco, hypertension, cholesterol, diabetes and alcohol abuse
14 DAYS, 6 HOURS

The impact, time trends and potential for prevention of premature deaths in Canada were assessed. There were almost 100,000 deaths before age 75 in Canada during 1986 resulting in over 1.7 million potential years of life lost (PYLL). The three leading broad disease categories responsible for PYLL were cancer, injuries/violence and cardiovascular disease. In both sexes, coronary heart disease, car accidents, lung cancer and perinatal conditions ranked in the top 5 specific diseases responsible for PYLL; breast cancer (females) and suicide (males) also ranked in the top 5 conditions. Over the period 1969 to 1986, death rates among persons less than age 75 increased for 3 conditions among females and 11 conditions among males. Lung cancer and brain cancer death rates increased in both sexes, chronic obstructive pulmonary disease death rates increased among females only and death rates for suicide and 8 types of cancer increased among males only. Over the same period, death rates declined for 37 discrete disease categories among both females and males including particularly large improvements for coronary heart disease, stroke, car accidents and perinatal conditions. An estimated 50,000 or over 50% of all premature deaths per year are preventable through control of smoking, hypertension, elevated serum cholesterol, diabetes and alcohol abuse. About 6,000 premature deaths are avoidable through improvements in medical care.

PMID: 2253155 [PubMed - indexed for MEDLINE]

In spite of the bias of this study ("An estimated 50,000 or over 50% of all premature deaths per year are preventable through control of smoking, etc"), a death is not avoided - at most, it is delayed - and "premature" refers to a theoretical average life span that does not apply to individuals. The theoretical gains in life span are absolutely pathetic - especially in consideration of what would be eliminated, and at what social cost. But the use of the word "avoid" appeals more effectively to emotions, with better results on the politicians that dispense public funds. Rational analysis is entirely bypassed.

What is the theoretical longevity gain for each Canadian, then? Even by pooling together all the "causes" and using the grand total: 1,170,000 years "lost" x the 365 days of the year = 427,050,000 days divided by 30 million Canadians = 14.24 days -- if we round it up.

ITALY

The gains in Italy are a little better (a bit more than two years); but to obtain that result cancer, AIDS and cardiovascular diseases -- and even traffic accidents -- must be

lumped together - THE IMPACT OF THE MAJOR CAUSES OF DEATH ON LIFE EXPECTANCY IN ITALY - Conti S, Farchi G, Masocco M, Toccaceli V, Vichi M. - Laboratory of Epidemiology and Biostatistics, Istituto Superiore di Sanita, Roma, Italy.
THE ENTIRE POPULATION
COMBINING THE REDUCTION OF CARDIOVASCULAR DISEASES, MALIGNANT TUMOURS, TRAFFIC ACCI-DENTS AND AIDS MORTALITY
2.27 years for men
2.16 years for women

BACKGROUND: This study aims to evaluate the contribu-tion of the reduction in major cardiovascular diseases (CVD), malignant neoplasms (MN), accidents and AIDS mortality to the gains in life expectancy observed during the decade 1985-1994, as well as to calculate and compare the potential gains due to the partial or total elimination of these causes. METHODS: Mortality data from the Italian Mortality Data Base were analysed by the method of de-composition of changes in life expectancy and the partial multiple decrement life table technique. RESULTS: In Italy, considering the decade 1985-1994, the gain in life expect-ancy at birth was 2.27 years for men and 2.16 for women. The major contribution to this increase was the reduction in CVD mortality followed by fewer deaths from accidents and MN. Conversely, AIDS caused a loss in the length of life of adults. Major potential gains in life expectancy at birth could be obtained by the elimination or even partial reduction of CVD and MN mortality. When working life (15-64 years) is considered, the relative importance of the causes changes. The elimination of accidents and AIDS would result in increased life expectancy longer than that associated with a 50% reduction in CVD. CONCLUSIONS: The findings of this study provide useful information which could contribute to a more effective allocation of re-sources for research activity and public health programmes.

PMID: 10597990 [PubMed - indexed for MEDLINE]

APPENDIX C

HAS EPA BEEN PROMOTING ONE BIG SECONDHAND SMOKE SCREEN?

By Joseph Perkins
Copyright 1998 Ventura County Star July 29, 1998

My neighborhood grill-and-ale house has banned smoking inside its premises since the first of the year. Those who choose to light up must do so in a designated smoking area outside. I must say, I like this arrangement.

I never cared to breathe the cigarette fumes of others. Nor did I like it when my clothes, my hair, even my skin reeked of tobacco smoke.

But having mentioned all this, I must also say that I do not like the reason my favorite watering hole went "smoke free." It was mandated by California state law, which took effect New Year's Day, banning smoking not only in restaurants, but also in bars.

And the pretext of this law was a 1993 study and declaration by the U.S. Environmental Protection Agency that secondhand smoke is a Class A carcinogen -- as hazardous as asbestos, benzene and radon -- and that it causes some 3,000 lung-cancer deaths a year.

Even folks like me who aren't cigarette smokers, who appreciate a smoke-free environment, suspected that the EPA's findings were politically motivated rather than based on sound science. And earlier this month, a federal judge in North Carolina arrived at the same conclusion.

"EPA publicly committed to a conclusion before research had begun," wrote U.S. District Court Judge William Osteen. Furthermore, the judge added, the regulatory agency violated federal law, the 1986 Radon Gas and Indoor Air Quality Research Act, in determining that secondhand smoke was a potent carcinogen.

The law requires that a broad-based panel be convened to make such determinations and that the panel include representatives of affected industries. However, the EPA deliberately excluded tobacco-industry representatives from its secondhand smoke panel.

Morover, wrote Osteen, the EPA "adjusted established procedure and scientific norms to validate the agency's public conclusions." In other words, the EPA dishonestly selected a small batch of studies that supported its desired conclusion -- that secondhand smoke causes lung cancer -- while ignoring a larger batch of studies that contradicted its finding.

Two of the studies the EPA ignored were actually sponsored by organizations that are anything but sympathetic to the tobacco industry. One study, funded by the National Cancer Institute, found that nonsmokers have no increased risk of lung cancer as a result of exposure to secondhand smoke during childhood, in the workplace or from living with a pack-a-day smoker for as many as 40 years.

Another study, conducted by the International Agency for Research on Cancer and funded by the World Health Organization, similarly concluded that secondhand smoke poses no significant health risk.

Despite these authoritative studies, despite Judge Osteen's ruling last week striking down the conclusion of the EPA's 1993 study, <u>the agency continues to deceive the public that secondhand is not merely a nuisance, but a proven health hazard</u>.

Moreover, wrote Osteen, the EPA "adjusted established procedure and scientific norms to validate the agency's public conclusions." In other words, <u>the EPA dishonestly selected a small batch of studies that supported its desired conclusion -- that secondhand smoke causes lung cancer -- while ignoring a larger batch of studies that contradicted its finding</u>.

But these same anti-smoking crusaders applauded the same judge last year -- a ruling to which the tobacco industry strenuously objected.

The issue here really is not so much about secondhand smoke. It's more about the corruption of science by the EPA for political purposes.

Joseph Perkins is a columnist for the San Diego Union-Tribune.

Environmental Tobacco Smoke and Coronary Heart Syndromes: Absence of an Association

By Gio Batta Gori

Ref: Regulatory Toxicology and Pharmacology 21, 281-295 (1995).

ABSTRACT

Concerns about possible cardiovascular and especially coronary effects of environmental tobacco smoke (ETS) derive from the reported effects of active smoking.

Numerous epidemiologic studies report that the **active** smoking of less than 10 cigarettes/day is **not**

associated with measurable risk of coronary heart disease (CHD). Thus, even assuming that ETS and MS have equivalent biological activities, conceivable ETS doses to nonsmokers are **far below apparent no-effect thresholds for active smoking.** Hence, it is no surprise that epidemiologic reports are **inconclusive** about a possible association of ETS exposure and CHD, some suggesting a slight elevation, others a reduction of risk. Often, the elevations reported are higher than the CHD risk values associated with active smoking. Such equivocations likely result from the presence of contrasting protective or aggravating confounders, of which more than 200 have been reported in the literature -- confounders that were not and could not be adequately controlled by any epidemiologic study. **By scientific standards, the weight of evidence continues to falsify the hypothesis that ETS exposure might be a CHD risk factor.**

* * *

INTRODUCTION

Several reviews have attempted to appraise the literature on environmental tobacco smoke (ETS) and coronary heart disease (CHD) (Glantz and Parmley, 1991; Taylor and Johnson, 1992; Steenland, 1992; Wells, 1994). In general these reviews have been **selective and conjectural** and have failed to account for the many pertinent considerations that a scientific evaluation requires. Although written by a long-time consultant to the tobacco industry, this present review strives for a comprehensive evaluation of available knowledge by avoiding assumptions and standing by the evidence.

In considering ETS as a possible CHD risk factor it will be useful to address what is known of the chemical, physical and biological comparability of ETS and the smoke that smokers inhale. Exposures and doses will then be compared in light of the no-observable adverse effect levels for active smoking and CHD, as reported in the literature. Finally, the epidemiologic studies of ETS exposure and possible CHD risk are evaluated against the background of numerous confounders, difficulties in establishing and measuring exposures, classification and other logical biases, statistical criteria of significance, and inferential conjectures from in vitro and in vivo experiments and clinical effects in humans.

ETS AND ACTIVE SMOKING

Mainstream smoke -- inhaled directly by smokers -- is concentrated and confined to the moist environment of mouth, throat, and lung. Its higher gas-phase concentrations favour larger respirable particles that condense and retain more water and volatiles. By contrast, ordinary ETS is over **100,000 times more diluted,** with much lower humidity and extremely low concentrations of volatiles. Evaporation is faster from ETS particles which -- within fraction of seconds from their generation -- attain sizes 50 to 100 times smaller in mass and volume than their mainstream counterparts. As ETS ages, it undergoes oxidative and photochemical transformation, polymerization from loss of water and volatiles, reactions with other environmental components, differential absorption to environmental surfaces, and other changes (NAS,1986; USSG,1986; USEPA,1992c; Guerin et al., 1987; Baker and Proctor, 1990). The reducing capacity and free radicals of MS are lost within minutes (Schmeltz et al., 1977,

Tanigawa et at.. 1994), and ETS is considerably less cytotoxic than inhaled MS (Sonnenfeld and Wilson,1987).

Of the several thousand components identified in mainstream smoke, only 100 or so have been detected in sidestream smoke under Field conditions, due to extreme dilutions. Because of even greater dilution, only about 20 ETS components have been identified directly under field conditions. In natural settings, most ETS components are below the sensitivity of current analytical capabilities (Guerin et al.,1987; Baker and Proctor.1990).

Compilers of ETS reports from the National Academy of Sciences (NAS, l986), the U.S. Surgeon General (USSG, 1986), and the Environmental Protection Agency (USEPA, 1992c) have been forced to infer the presence of ETS components **by proxy,** based on the composition of the sidestream smoke from which ETS primarily derives.

Nominally, then, ETS and mainstream smoke may share some components, but their chemical and physical differences are substantial. Moreover, the presence of most ETS components can only be postulated because they are beyond material detection. Also, the chemical and biologic reactivity of ETS is less than that for the MS that active smokers inhale, because of the loss of free radicals, other quenching, and absorption Losses during dilution and aging.

ESTIMATING ETS EXPOSURE

Estimates of exposure to other ETS components are even more problematic because of the numerous sources external to ETS. For instance, plasma concentrations of volatile organics in nonsmokers appear to be as much as two-thirds of the corresponding levels in active smokers (Angerer et al., 1992; Brugnone et al, 1992; Perbellini et al., 1988) -- an indication of significant sources other than tobacco combustion (Ritcher et al., 1994; Ong et al., 1994).

By utilizing surrogate sidestream smoke values, conceivable ETS exposure has been compared with current federal standards of permissible occupational exposure to several smoke components. Considering an unventilated room of 100 m3 (3533 cubic feet), the number of cigarettes that would have to be burned before reaching official threshold limit values varies among **1170** for methylchlorided to **13,300** for benzene to **222,000** for benzo(a) pyrene to **1,000,000** for toluene (Gori and Mantel, 1991).

For the average ETS-exposed individual, this estimate translates into an annual dose equivalent to far less than the mainstream RSP of <u>one cigarette evenly dispersed over a 12-month period</u> (Gori and Mantel, 1991).

COULD MINUTE ETS EXPOSURES POSE A HEALTH RISK?

Because direct measurements of the biologic activities, exposures, and doses of ETS are so problematic, initial attempts have inferred ETS-linked health risks by arithmetic derivation from the APPARENT risk associated with active smoking. However, this approach has been controversial.

Moreover, epidemiologic studies of active smoking give evidence of **No-Observable-Adverse-Effect-**levels (NOAELs), namely that at low daily consumption of cigarettes the epidemiologic risks associated with certain diseases become nonsignificant (Gori, 1976; Gori and Mantel, 1991). No- effect observations at comparatively high doses are also routinely reported in experimental animal exposure to whole smoke or its fractions. In a recent evaluation of smoking and health issues, the Congressional Research Service of the Library of Congress stated:

"The existence of an exposure treshold for disease onset below which many passive smokers fall in not implausible. Most organisms have the capacity to cleanse themselves of some level of contaminants. It is for this reason that public policy usually does not insist that every unit of air or water pollution be removed from the environment... In fact, strongly non-linear relationships in which health effects rise with the square of the exposure, and more, have been found with respect to active smoking (see Surgeon General's Report, 1989, p. 44). Were these relationships projected backwards to construct the lower (unknown) portion of the health effect/physical damage function, the observed relationship might lead researchers a priori to expect no empirical relationship. Thus, the issue raised by the potential break in the causative chain is whether researchers should expect to find a significant relationship between passive smoking and health effects." (Gravelle and Zimmermann, 1994, p. 45).

ETS AND POSSIBLE CHD RISK FACTORS IN HUMANS

Significantly, studies report that the aborted fetuses from smoking mothers have **40% less chromosomal abnormalities** than fetuses from nonsmoking mothers (Kline et al., 1993), while other studies report that maternal smoking is associated with a much decreased risk of mongoloid retardation or Down syndrome (Kline et al., 1993; Cuckle et al., 1990).

Studies of human lung cancer tissues found that serum cotinine levels and adduct levels were not correlated and could detect adducts only in 7 of 38 individual tumour samples (Shields et al., 1993) DNA adducts of aromatic hydrocarbons in lymphocytes were not found to correlate with smoking habits (van Schooten et al., 1992; Grzybowska et al., 1993). DNA adducts **were at similar levels in sperm cells of smokers and nonsmokers,** a finding of interest given the intense DNA replication in spermatogenesis (Gallagher et al., 1993). Equal similarities were reported for DNA adducts of cervix tissues (King et al., 1994).

ETS, thrombus formation. Hypotheses have proposed that increased blood-clotting capacity may explain the association of heavy smoking and cardiovascular events. However the Framingham study reports an absence of cardiovascular risks for smokers of 1-10 cigarettes/day, consonant with an immaterial change in mean fibrogen (about 1%) in smokers of less than one pack of cigarettes/day (Kannel et al., 1987). It has been suggested that two eicosanoids, prostacyclin and tromboxane A2 are altered in smoking, but studies indicate **no change in smokers of less that 10- 15 cigarettes/day** (Wennalm et al., 1991). The large Koupio prospective study in Finland found a correlation of plasma fibrinogen levels with several psychosocial and socioeconomic variables, **but not with smoking** (Kubisz et al., 1994). Vicari et al., (1988) measured several thrombotic factors and found **no differences due to active smoking**. Haire et al. (1988) found no change in fibrinolytic activity after active smoking. Yamashita et al (1988) **found no effect of smoking on platelet aggregation**. Handley and Teather (1974) and Barbashet al. (1993, 1994) give an indication that smoking may protect against thromboembolic compilations after myocardial infarction and surgery. Similar results were reported by Pollack and Evans (1978). The Arteriosclerosis Risk in Communities Study of 15,800 men and women in the United States found that **smoking was positively associated with levels of Antithrombin III, a major anticoagulant factor** (Conlan et al.,1994). **Some studies that suggest differently have been flawed or misinterpreted.**

ETS, cholesterol, lipidemias, and hypertension.

The Cardiovascular Health Study Collaborative Research Group reports that in a cohort of 5201 men and women over 65 years of age, **cigarette smoking was a negative predictor of blood pressure, confirming a number of prior reports** (Tell et al., 1994).

The massive WHO-MONICA study actually "showed a strong negative association between regular smoking and high cholesterol in the male populations and a strong negative association between regular smoking and high blood pressure in female populations" (MONICA, 1994). Well known is the so-called "French paradox," whereby the French population shows **55% less CHDs** than the rest of the population surveyed in the MONICA project, despite experiencing high levels of cigarette smoking, hypertension, and total cholesterol (Renaud and de Longeril, 1993). The Helsinki Ageing Study reports a **sight inverse association of active smoking and aortic valve degeneration** in the elderly (Lindroos et al., 1994). In China, coronary mortality is **some 10 times less frequent than in Germany,** although the prevalence of smoking is **70% in China versus 37% in Germany.** Total cholesterol, however, is much higher in German than in Chinese subjects (Stehle et al., 1991).

These considerations tell that the active smoking of less than 10 cigarettes/day or ETS exposures are unlikely to adversely influence lipidemic Coronary Heart Disease risk factors. As such, they support the notion of No-Observable-Adverse-Effect-Levels for active smoking and cardiovascular diseases. In fact, the National Cholesterol Education Program only lists smoking over 10 cigarettes/day as possible CHD risk factor (NCEP, 1988).

A Fraudulent Study

RE: Cigarette smoking and progression of atherosclerosis, the Atherosclerosis Risk in Communities (ARIC) Study. By George Howard, DrPh; Lynne E Wagenknecht, DrPh; Gregory L Burke, MD, MS; Ana Diez-Roux, PhD; Gregory W. Evans, MS; Paul McGovern, PhD; F Javier Nieto, MD, PhD; Gretna S Tell, PhD; for the ARIC investigators. Journal of the American Medical Association 1998 Jan 14;279(2):119-124.

AND: What's so passive about passive smoking? Secondhand smoke as a cause of atherosclerotic disease. (Editorial re Howard et al). By Rachel M Werner and Thomas A Pearson, MD, PhD. Journal of the American Medical Association 1998 Jan 14;279(2):157-158.

ALSO MEDIA ACCOUNTS OF THE ABOVE: Study Probes Second-Hand Smoke. By Lindsey Tanner, AP - Chicago. AP 13-Jan-1998 20:19 EST REF5582. Ex-Smokers May Have Irreversible D amage to Arteries, Wake Forest Study Shows. By Robert Conn, Mark Wright & Jim Steele, Wake Forest University Baptist Medical Center. PR Newswire 1998 Jan 13, 1737.

AHA Says Study on Secondhand Smoke Supports ...U.S. Newswire 1998 OTC 01/14 0002.

Scary evidence of smoking's danger. Study finds damage to arteries never heals. By Brigid Schulte, Knight-Ridder Newspapers. Wisconsin State Journal 1998 Wed Jan 14, p A2.

Let Us Have the Real Truth

February 9, 2000

The latest world health statistics show that the world's sickest countries are firstly the US then New Zealand. Both these countries have the most draconian anti-smoking agenda, second only to that of the Third Reich.

The healthiest country in the world and the lowest infant death rate is held by Japan, who also oddly enough has the highest smoking rate.

Italy another country envied for its longevity has a similarly high smoking rate.

This revelation was made recently on radio and newspapers and still the zealot's blame the ills of these countries on smoking, which by the way it has halved since the agenda against smoking began.

No one will answer the question I ask on this, none in the media will even listen when I ask. They don't even try to investigate how it can be that the US and New Zealand infant death rate is the highest in the world, yet the smoking rate has dropped -- and why the Japanese have almost eliminated cot death yet they smoke like chimneys.

Why has the asthma rate in New Zealand tripled but they still continue to lambast the smoker for this? After all, the smoking rate (they keep telling us) is dropping and because of the draconian Smoke-free laws asthma sufferers are less exposed to the scumbag smoker.

Why once upon a time when smokers smoked in offices and building the asthma rates were a third lower?

Lung cancer rates have doubled over the period of the anti-smoking agenda -- please explain. Why do non-smokers get lung cancer?

Why did the World health Organization hide ten full years of scientific research telling them that <u>passive smoking **DOESN'T** cause lung cancer</u>? Yet they continue to say it does.

Why did the US bother to get Judge Osteen to look into the work done on ETS if after his extensive study <u>striking down the EPA junk science findings on ETS</u> they then proceeded to ignore it?

All I ask is for the media to be investigative on this issue. The smoker and the tobacco industry have been turned into the lowest of life forms based on a lie. I ask: who is fibbing now?

Joy Faulkner
Founder Smokers Of the World Unite
President FORCES INTERNATIONAL (NZ)
Spokesman on Tobacco and Alcohol Libertarians

APPENDIX D

THE SOCIAL AND ECONOMIC IMPACT OF TOBACCO

Introduction

Tobacco's influence on social and economic issues dates back several centuries. Decade-to-decade growth in tobacco consumption is virtually uninterrupted -- since 1556 when explorer Andre` Thevert brought tobacco from Brazil to his native France (among tobacco's earliest points of entry into Europe).

Ongoing trade activities between France and various South American settlers were soon established -- making tobacco one of Brazil's most profitable export crops of that time.

Today in the developing nations, farmers find numerous incentives for growing tobacco.

Among them: stability of the world-wide demand for the crop; relative ease in transporting tobacco; and tobacco's profitability when compared with other crops.

These factors, and others, make tobacco one of the most appealing cash crops in nations where immediate return on investment is essential for the farmers' survival. (In a later section, we will examine replacing tobacco with other crops.)

The socio-economic influence of tobacco farming extends beyond the immediate interest of the farmer, reaching out to the farming communities and beyond -- affecting the economies of entire nations.

While data regarding tobacco's expansive global appeal as a valuable farm commodity is impressive and worthy of discussion here, it is equally important to focus on tobacco's socio-economic impact within individual nations, as well as within the farm communities of those nations.

Profitability for growers

World consumption of tobacco increased by seven per cent from 1992 to 1995, and is projected to increase by an additional five to seven percent by the turn of the century.

This steady demand for the crop and relative stability of the world tobacco market prices make tobacco one of the most appealing cash crops for farmers in developing regions. In these areas, farmers cannot afford to invest in crops that bring unsteady prices or unpredictable demand. By producing tobacco, farmers can effectively increase the level of cash income necessary for acquiring inputs for production of food crops.

The profitability of tobacco reaches well beyond the farm, as economic activity does not occur in isolation. Farmers who reap a profit from their tobacco crop will, in turn, sped a portion of the money on various goods and services for themselves and their families, as well as for their farm.

In Zimbabwe, which exports 98 percent of its tobacco, the crop has a 'multiplier effect' on the local economy estimated to be 4.3 times the cost of production. For example, a kilogram of tobacco which cost Z\$7.88 to produce was found to generate Z\$33.84 within the local economy. [6]

Employment: An Indispensable Benefit of Tobacco

No other crop creates as much employment per hectare of cultivated land as tobacco [7]. This fact, alone, paints a clear picture of tobacco's socio-economic impact in developing nations. Estimates suggest that is workers' families, seasonal workers and landless labourers are included, some 33 million people are currently employed through tobacco growing and early stages of processing. If all tobacco-related industries and processes are included, the figure is at least 100 million - nearly 90 percent of whom are in developing nations. [9]

By comparison, only about 1.6 million people are involved in the cultivation of maize or sugar cane.

Despite technological progress, tobacco cultivation (for large and small farms, alike) has remained one of the most labour-intensive operations in all of agriculture. (For example, the production of flue-cured tobacco in Tanzania requires 533 man days per hectare, compared with 217 man days per hectare for rice, the next most labour- intensive crop.) Generally, tobacco is a crop not readily mechanised except in richer countries and on larger farms. Women, in particular, and unskilled labourers who would otherwise have a little chance of employment are therefore able to earn a living. This is especially important in developing nations, where rural employment can be scarce.

The employment created by tobacco growing extends beyond the farm fields. The tobacco must be sorted, stored, auctioned, processed, packaged for dispatch, transported to the ports and loaded on ships. In nations where tobacco growing is prevalent, an extensive industry of processing establishments, auction houses, warehousing firms, carriers, packers, transhipment companies and insurers -- right down to local production and distribution centres -- has sprouted up around the growing process.

Jobs created from these industries are especially important in nations where the agricultural sector is already depressed. The World Health Organization (WHO) even acknowledges that in such nations it may be difficult to find alternative employment for those previously employed in the agricultural sector. [9]

In numerous developing nations, such as Tanzania and Malawi in south central Africa, the vast employment created on tobacco farms has curbed migration from rural areas to the over-populated cities -- a problem common in developing nations. In Malawi, it was estimated in 1987 by the Ministry of Labour that nearly one third of total paid employment in that nation was derived from the tobacco industry. The economic impact of tobacco in nations such as Malawi cannot be disputed -- even by the WHO, which has reported that tobacco is the 'backbone' of that nation's economy, noting that tobacco exports in 1990 accounted for almost 70 per cent of total income from exports. [10] In such nations, it can be safely assumed that any reduction in tobacco farming (even if it were replaced by other less labour-intensive crops) would harm the nations' economies and probably lead to increased poverty.

In Thailand, where a predominantly agricultural based society is transforming into an industrial base, farming still accounts for about two thirds of the nation's employment. And it is estimated that in the tobacco growing sectors of Thailand, more than one million people are employed full or part-time by way of this industry.

As an agricultural commodity that helps employ at least 33 million people in the production process, tobacco's positive socio-economic contributions are indisputable.

Tobacco's Contribution to Foreign Exchange

Developing nations have always relied heavily on the export of agricultural products as one of their few viable sources of foreign exchange earnings. And indeed, tobacco makes significant contributions to the economy of many of these developing nations through foreign exchange receipt and sales on the international market. In 1987, the world's developing countries received more than US$1.7 billion in foreign exchange receipts from tobacco sales on the international market. [11] In the absence of any comparable alternatives, government continue to regards tobacco exports as a lucrative and reliable source of funding for their economic ad social development plans.

For example, in Brazil, the Dominican Republic, India and Tanzania, tobacco contributes to about five percent of total agricultural exports. For the Republic of Korea and Turkey, it rises to about 12 percent, and in Malawi and Zimbabwe, tobacco export earnings provide some 56 percent and 47 percent, respectively. [12] Indeed for the latter two countries, tobacco provides 74 percent of foreign exchange earnings in Malawi and over 30 percent in Zimbabwe.

Tobacco's high degree of price stability also enhances its foreign exchange capacity. Widely fluctuating world prices for other farm products present problems for many developing nations. Over the years, the stability of tobacco exports earnings consistently out-performs that for a host of other export commodities -- including sugar, coffee, tea and rice.

Government Revenue From Tobacco

Historically, tobacco has been one of the most heavily taxed consumer products in the world, consequently creating much-needed government revenue. In nations of all sizes and socio-economic standing, tobacco is often taxed at the local and national level. While specific tax policies vary from country to country, taxes on tobacco are often levied throughout the various stages of its production, distribution and sales -- i.e. levied on farmers based on the amount of tobacco grown; on the importers and exporters; on the manufacturers that purchase the leaf; and on the consumer of tobacco products at the time of purchase. It is likely that many of those who are employed by the various sectors of tobacco production have concerns about whether their product may be overtaxed.

In an era when some tobacco opponents propose additional taxes on tobacco products merely to curtail the consumer demand (i.e. 'taxing tobacco out of existence'), tobacco growers are understandably wary discussing the benefits of taxation. But numerous governments of rich and poor nations alike rely on tobacco taxes as a significant source of revenue. And while tobacco farmers, manufacturers, importers/ exporters and consumers may want explicit limitations on taxation, the fact remains that these taxes greatly enhance tobacco's socio-economic importance to many nations.

"NOT ONLY IS TOBACCO AN IMPORTANT ECONOMIC COMMODITY, BUT FOR A NUMBER OF COUNTRIES IT IS AN IMPORTANT SOURCE OF INCOME AND FOREIGN CURRENCY."

Pakistan - 40 percent of all government excise taxes and 10 percent of total government revenue are via tobacco.

Philippines - Excise taxes on tobacco account for about 20 percent of all government revenues. Brazil - Tobacco taxation represents nearly six percent of all tax revenues.

Malawi - In 1991, income tax paid by growers, merchants and their employees amounted to the equivalent of US$40 million or 11 percent of the total tax revenues. [14] The remarkable internal revenue produced by tobacco taxes enables governments to better serve their citizens through various services -- such as enhanced education and health care. Education is an important catalyst to the socio-economic development of any nation. And in tobacco-producing regions of a number of countries, revenue from tobacco production and consumption contribute to the educational need of rural communities through construction of facilities and employment of teachers. Similarly, in developing areas, governments often struggle to provide adequate health care for their citizens. Tobacco produced taxes often make the difference in providing medical facilities, staff and medication accessible to all the population.

Conclusion

Tobacco's revenue-producing attributes cannot be denied. Expenditures undertaken by tobacco growers, their families and seasonal workers have favourable economic effects in the individual farming communities, as well as positive impact throughout the various nations.

Profitable tobacco farmers play a role in enhancing the agricultural infrastructure necessary for the growth of other traditional food crops. Tobacco profits lead to the financing of schools, health services, roads, water supplies and environmental improvement initiatives.

In many nations, tobacco facilitates capital formation for other industries, including transportation, finance, construction, retail and wholesale trading and manufacturing. Shops, markets and small businesses that cater to the needs of farm workers and their families benefit from tobacco production. All these enterprises would be adversely affected by the tobacco farmers' loss of income.

The Strong, Stable Market

Demand for tobacco continues to steadily increase. To meet the increases in tobacco consumption, world production of tobacco increased by seven percent from 1992 to 1995 -- with the largest increase seen in developing nations such as Indonesia, China and Zimbabwe. In developed nations, growth during this period was about one percent.

Simply, with the increases in tobacco consumption and production, it is difficult for tobacco growers to consider making substantial changes in their crop selection -- for as long as the demand for the product exists, production will continue. Given the continued stability in the tobacco market, reduction of the resources devoted to the production of tobacco in one country would only result in an increase of production in other countries.

Tobacco farmers throughout the world find comfort in the relative stability of the world tobacco market prices. Virtually all studies of tobacco price stability, when compared with price stability of other crops, show that farmers' confidence in tobacco is justified. The World Health Organization has acknowledged i its writing that other crops than can potentially give high returns (such as fruits and vegetables) "have limited potential because of market constraints and unstable prices." [15] And according to the United Nations Conference on Trade and Development (UNCTAD), between 1984 and 1993 tobacco prices were two, three, and four time more stable than those of wheat, tea and sugar, respectively. In fact, with the exception of beef, tobacco was the most stable of over 30 commodities. [16] This factor, when linked to continuing market outlets, give farmers far greater security than most other crops.

The stability of price levels is of great importance, especially in the case of producers in developing areas who cannot afford the financial risk of investing in crops that provide unsteady prices from year to year. While fluctuating commodity prices may be nothing more than an occasional distraction for many farmers in developed regions, a sudden drop in prices could easily lead to dreadful economic hardship -- even starvation -- in the least developed regions.

Also, in developing nations some crops are well-known for their insufficient marketing and support infrastructure -- often leading to long delays between sale of the crop and payment. This is an important drawback for farmers, especially when high interest rates are considered. And tobacco farmers are accustomed to trading practices which ensure rapid payment for their crops.

As discussed previously, no other crop creates as much employment per hectare of cultivated land as tobacco. The nature of tobacco crops requires meticulous "hands-on" labour. Millions of unskilled labourers, who otherwise would be most likely unemployed, earn a living in tobacco cultivation. Tobacco's high labour requirements have been instrumental in stemming the flow of under-employed and unemployed people from rural to urban areas. Therefore, tobacco in developing nations is often seen as a means to partially alleviate the socio-economic and political problems associated with surplus labour.

In the debate regarding alternative crops, only tobacco can boast such a tremendous influence on employment.

Tobacco's ability to grow well in climates and soils unsuitable for other crops gives it an immediate edge over many alternatives. In many developing nations, the soil is too poor and offers too few nutrients for most other food crops. As a hardy and sun-loving plant, tobacco can tolerate a wide variation in rainfall patterns while still yielding a commercial crop -- unlike cereals or soybeans which cannot be grown in such extreme conditions.

In regions where fragmented farmland and widely dispersed field are prevalent -- regardless of those nations' socio- economic levels -- tobacco growing is a sensible choice, as adequate mechanisation for alternatives may bi impractical or impossible to introduce. This is true in the tobacco hotbeds of the southeast United States, as well as in Greece, Italy and numerous smaller, developing nations. [17] Also, most of the farms that grow tobacco, especially in the Far East consist of relatively small plots of land, as few crops can match tobacco's per hectare profitability, and this provides for a family substinence.

About 25 percent of tobacco produced world-wide is internationally traded. Although the US is still a leading exporter (especially of high-quality flue-cured tobacco), the developing countries have caught up considerably. These nations regard tobacco as an indispensable source of foreign exchange, bringing in more exports of other commodities. For example, in Zimbabwe -- the major tobacco producer in south central Africa -- nearly all of its tobacco is exported. In fact, tobacco shipments amount to up to 60 percent of the nation's total agricultural exports. About half of Thailand's tobacco crop is exported.

The steady world-wide demand on tobacco is not the only reason for its role as an important source of foreign exchange. In developing countries, the cost of transporting tobacco for export is considerably less compared to other agricultural products. Tobacco's high value/weigh ratio allows it to absorb costs of long journeys. It weighs relatively little, requires comparatively less transportation space than other exports such as most vegetables, fruits and flower. It is also considerably less perishable.

In many tobacco producing countries, national growers associations actively advise members on the growing and marketing of other crops. This helps growers to maximize their income from rotational farming. For example, AFUBRA in Brazil has demonstration farms which show how best to produce maize and black beans as well as tobacco.

Indeed, one of the most important obstacles to extensive growth in alternative crop production is the difficulty in transporting the highly perishable goods to market. Many developing countries do not have adequate infrastructure for rapid movement of such goods to seaports or airports. High rates for air freight and low capacity, along with meagre selection of export destinations, make air transportation difficult.

Where complementary crops are grown, the lack of custom-built transport for carrying highly perishable produce, plus the high cost of air freight, tends to force exporters to concentrate on premium products such as strawberries, asparagus and cut flowers. Some of these premium commodities offer potential financial returns in excess of those generated by tobacco. But they also require an enormous (and often prohibitive) initial capital investment, and pose higher risks. They are expensive to grow, transport and market.

Sometimes, deciduous tree fruit and citrus are mentioned as possible alternatives for the tobacco crop. But growers would realize no income for several years after the initial investment, until the trees have reached the bearing stage. In most developing nations, farmers simply cannot afford such a wait.

In many nations, crops like tea, coffee and sugar are inhibited by internal quotas, which largely determine how much a country can produce. In any case, these products are already grown extensively and, should additional production ever be required, it would almost certainly be on existing estates and plantations -- where the land, equipment, labour and skills are already available.

Tobacco and Food Supply

In view of the need for increased food supply within many developing nations, some final comments should be made regarding the claim that excessive production of tobacco is interfering with production of much-needed food crops.

First, supported by the information presented in this document, the suggestion top replace tobacco with food crops simply cannot be supported. Certainly, the need for increased food supplies in particular areas may, at times, be substantial. But factors other than tobacco farming must be considered when analyzing the causes.

In many developing nations (India and Malawi, for example) problems regarding food supply are most markedly related to political inequities and inadequate infrastructure. Generally, crop losses due to inadequate or insufficient storage and transport can reach 40 percent of the quantity harvested.

A study of nearly 1,000 farms in 1996 by AFUBRA, the Brazilian tobacco growers' association, found that tobacco provides an average annual income of US$8,000 for every family that grow the crop. Parallel crops (grow in rotation with tobacco) bring an extra US$2,000, The survey also revealed that a farmer has to grow 9 hectares of corn to equal the income from 1 hectare of tobacco. [19]

More importantly, tobacco's far-reaching socio-economic impact in developing nations simply cannot be overlooked. Tobacco, compared with other cash crops, offers a high degree of security of income. Earnings are paid out immediately after sale. This provides farmers with the necessary cash for investment in other areas of agriculture as well. Often, a substantial portion of a nation's staple foods -- maize, beef, wheat, soybean, etc. -- are produced by tobacco farms. And, as discussed previously, most of the world's tobacco farms are on relatively small areas of land -- where high profitability per hectare is essential.

A study in the Migori District of Kenya examining the economic influence of tobacco cultivation on the production of food supported two conclusions: First, tobacco had no significant negative effect on production of food crops; second, tobacco was the most profitable per unit of land of the four enterprises examined -- tobacco, beans, maize, diary. [20] By producing tobacco,, farmers would most effectively increase the level of cash income vital for acquiring inputs for food crop production. In Zimbabwe, over 80 percent of diversification has been undertaken by tobacco farmers who have the capital resources necessary.

Conclusion

Without question, tobacco is an important export commodity and a substantial source of foreign exchange for many developing nations. It is also a major generator of rural employment and provides the means for peasant farmers to break away from mere substinence agriculture. Tobacco cultivation utilises more labour than most other crops. Its labour-intensity is instrumental in stemming the flow of under-employed and unemployed people from rural to urban areas.

It has also been noted that cultivation of tobacco represents only a modest use of agricultural land. Therefore, the argument that tobacco should be replaced by food crops is irrelevant. In fact, most data indicates that tobacco production assists in facilitating the spread of improved crop husbandry techniques for the production of other crops. Tobacco's ability to grow in soils and climates that are not conductive to other food products also negates the argument for replacing tobacco with food staples.

In the foreseeable future, tobacco farmers are not likely to responds to calls to cease production of such sustainable crop. Farmers will continue to invest in tobacco production as long as consumer demand for tobacco products exists at current of higher levels, and as long as they can be assured that their crops will sell quickly and profitably. Equally as important, as prudent agricultural businessmen, they will invest in new opportunities as they arise.

References

1. Chollat-Tracquet, C. (1996) Evaluating Tobacco Control Activities, World Health Organization, Geneva, p. 32.

2. ITGA (1996) Tobacco -- a major world crop, ITGA Issues Paper No. 2, East Grinstead, England.

3. US Department of Agriculture (1994) World Tobacco Situation Report, Foreign Agriculture Service.

4. Reuters, April 18, 1996.

5. UN ECOSOC (1994) Annex II - Position Paper of the Food and Agriculture Organization of the United Nations on Tobacco Cultivation, Multisectoral Collaboration on Tobacco or Health UN Economic and Social Council, 21 June 1994, p. 23.

6. Rooney, M & Ellis, M. (1994) Zimbabwe Tobacco - An Important Economic Impact Study, unpublished paper, Harare, p. 2.

7. Reemstma (1995) Tobacco -- Driving Forces for Economic Development.

8. Chollat-Traquet, C. (1996) Evaluating Tobacco Control Activities, World Health Organization, Geneva, p. 32-36

10. ibid, p. 33.

11. FAO (1989 The Economic Significance of Tobacco, FAO Economic and Social Development Paper 85, Rome.

12. ibid.

13. Chollat-Traquet, C. op. cit., p. 38.

14. Agro-Economic Services Ltd and Tabacosmos Ltd, The employment, tax revenue and wealth that the tobacco industry creates. London, 1987, Table A 3.6.

15. Chollat-Tracquet, C. op. cit., p. 33.

16. World Bank (1994) Commodity Markets and the Developing Countries, Washington.

17. Patchett, D. Alternatives to Tobacco Tobacco Forum, ITGA, Col 2, No. 2.

18. AFUBRA (1996) Brazilian Tobacco Grower Profile, Santa Cruz do Sul.

20. Oyugi, L.A., Mukhebi, A.W. and Mwangi, W.M. (1987) The Impact of Cash Cropping on Food Production: A Case Study of Tobacco and Maize in Migari Division, South Nyanza District of Kenya. East African Economic Review, Volume 3, No. 1.

Bibliography

International Tobacco Growers' Association, East Grinstead, England:

(1990) Tobacco in the Developing World.

(1992 and 1993) Tobacco farming: Sustainable alternatives, vol. !, 1992 and vol. 2, 1993.

(1992) The economic significance of tobacco growing in Central and Southern Africa.

(1994) Tobacco Trade or Aid?

(1996) Tobacco Growers -- Issues Papers.

Campbell, J.S. (1994) Tobacco and the Environment, CORESTA Congress Paper, Harare Chilowa, W.

(1993) The significance of tobacco in the economy of Malawi, University of Malawi, Centre for Social Research, Blantyre.

FAO (1990) Tobacco: supply, demand and trade projections 1995 and 2000, FAO Economic and Social Development Paper 86, Rome

APPENDIX E

<u>FROM THE CIGAR BARON</u>

Dr. Marc Schneiderman and the Internet Cigar Group

The following summary was posted by the FAQ's author, cigarbaron@aol.com (Cigar Baron), who is Paraphrasing Wynder and Mabuchi, 1972.

(1) Heavy cigar and pipe smoking is associated with the development of lung cancer.

(2) Cigar and pipe smokers have a lower risk of lung cancer than the cigarette smoker. We believe this finding to relate to differences in inhalation practices and to the age at which smoking began.

(3) The lower risk of lung cancer for Jewish males does not apply for cigar and pipe smoking, indicating the lower overall risk of lung cancer for Jewish males to relate to the lesser usage of cigarettes rather than to constitutional factors.

(4) The age of male lung cancer patients who have smoked only cigars and pipes is older than for cigarette smokers, possibly reflecting an older age at the start of smoking and longer life expectancy of cigar and pipe smokers as compared to cigarette smokers, or a lesser deposition of tobacco smoke in the respiratory tract of cigar and pipe smokers due to the fact that they are predominantly non-inhalers. It is also possible that this

358 / The Health Benefits of Tobacco

reflects the secular changes in smoking habits that has taken place in the general population.

(5) While light cigars (one to two a day) or pipe smoking (one to four a day) does not appear to be associated with an increased risk of lung cancer, heavier cigar and pipe smokers need to realize that their risk for lung cancer as well as for other types of cancer and diseases is quite appreciable.

Essentially all major articles had some procedural flaw. The conclusions however all reflect the above two statements, and continually be reconfirmed. My personal feeling is that 2-3 cigars per day, not inhaled, pose no significant health threat.

There are no studies that implicate "light" cigar smoke with an increased health risk. However, cigars certainly are implicated in lung and other forms of cancer, and once you smoke 5+ a day, the risks become substantial. We cannot consider cigars benign

The Cigar/Health FAQ is available on the Web at
http://www.cigargroup.com/faq/health

Tobacco and Marijuana:
Let us stop insulting truth and common sense

June 19, 2002

The sad news (assuming it's true) that smoking is now banned in 60 percent of Canadian homes demonstrates, if any more proof is needed, that any lie (no matter how outrageous) which has enough money behind it can become a truth – especially when health authorities such as the Canadian Ministry of Health become the instruments of the pharmaceutical multinationals. I am talking about the passive smoke fraud, of course, and the false belief that passive smoke represents a sizeable danger to the health of people.

But the "suggestions" of the self-serving poll (reported by Mr. McKenzie of the Canadian Press on May 26, 2002) implemented and financed by those very same who lie about smoking for a living, are not really the issue of this piece. The issue here is that Mr. Sweanor, counsel for the Non-Smokers' Rights Association in Canada, goes beyond any limit of decency with the statement: "...But now, it's at the stage where smoking in the house is generally seen as something like 'Do you mind if I defecate on your floor'?" But then he surpasses himself with this breathtaking assertion: "There's no question that cigarette-smoking is massively more harmful than marijuana. The reality is that marijuana is not killing people and tobacco is killing 45,000 a year."

Reality? Come on, David: I know that the addiction to public money has really got to your head, but this is really too much! Let's put aside the fact that you cannot prove that ONE single death is caused uniquely by smoking – and that you can't even quantify the contribution of tobacco to one single death on earth, because it is impossible. Thus the 45,000-deaths figure means absolutely nothing.

Let us talk about marijuana instead. Like too many antismokers, Mr. Sweanor suffers from conveniently severe schizophrenia about this drug. The schizophrenia goes just about like this: smoking tobacco is baaaad -- but smoking cannabis is not. Hmmm... let's see: don't they both burn organic materials? Isn't it true that in joints there is often a large amount of tobacco? Isn't it true that marijuana emits a very thick, irritating passive smoke that can be smelled from blocks away? I find it absolutely absurd that people who call themselves "anti-prohibition" (on marijuana) often support prohibition of tobacco, and are "disturbed" by tobacco smoking! Perhaps this is a generational revenge, going back to the times when mummy and daddy, cigs dangling from their lips, were giving their baby boomer progeny hell for being stoned all the time. Clearly, too many of my generation (the hippie one) never grew up and out of the Sixties. They are still protesting that ma and pa had it all wrong, but now, unfortunately, they have power -- or perhaps they have smoked so many joints that they are permanently stoned.

Let me say upfront that I am a real anti-prohibition type. I am against the war on drugs and the war on tobacco. Junk science mortality aside, I believe that the individual is sovereign, and he can do with his body what he sees fit (even when it kills him), and that the state has no right to intervene; finally, I am a strong supporter of intelligent drug legalization, that would shut down the factories of crime, and ensure the quality of drugs and delivery devices, thus preventing countless real deaths due to OD and AIDS, which unlike the computer-generated statistical associations for tobacco can be properly documented and pinned down as to causality.

With that qualification, no one can say that I am an anti-marijuana type. Smoke it and be happy! On the other hand, individuals like Sweanor truly make me sick, because (once again) they intentionally mislead people to advance an agenda, which clearly wouldn't mind seeing the marijuana prohibition swapped with the tobacco prohibition, and advancing that agenda with the flat and absurd statement that tobacco kills people while cannabis does not. Do you smoke joints, Mr. Sweanor? Smoking a joint today seems to be the politically correct way to smoke and be "in," and "acceptable. The very cheats who tell us that tobacco kills millions can smoke marijuana and get away with it by even calling it "therapeutic". *Look at this, mom and pop, I have done it! Roll in your grave with your cigarettes, you bastards – I am smoking a joint and you can't stop me anymore, see?*

Let us touch upon how things really are with cannabis:

Marijuana is fat-soluble, and it stays in the body for weeks, unlike alcohol, which is water-soluble and leaves the body in hours. It is a complex mixture of over 400 chemicals and over 60 cannabinoids, (missing in tobacco) including delta-9-tetrahydrocannabinol (THC), the main psychoactive ingredient. [1] THC, the marijuana ingredient associated with health "benefits", is currently available in pill form as Marinol TM, and it can be administered in known and precise doses, unlike smoked marijuana. [2] For each medical condition for which smoked marijuana is claimed to be beneficial, there are other drugs available that are superior to marijuana. [3] But we don't wanna hear about that, right? It would remove the real reason we want people to believe that cannabis has unique therapeutic characteristics: because we like to smoke it, and get stoned!

One study based on instrumental quantitative analysis of toxic components of cannabis smoke found that smoking a "joint" of marijuana caused over 10 times as much lung damage as smoking one cigarette. [4] Where did lung cancer go, dear anti-tobacco/pro-marijuana activists? Shouldn't we be at least 10 times as concerned about marijuana as we are about tobacco, assorted ministries of health and antitobacco freaks? Marijuana has not been shown to be a safe and effective drug in lowering intraocular pressure and preventing optic nerve damage for glaucoma patients. To maintain a low intraocular pressure with marijuana, a person would have to smoke a joint every 1 to 2 hours, 10 to 12 joints a day, and 4,000 a year. [5] That would put the toxic chemical intake at an equivalent of 100 to 144 cigarettes a day (or 36, 000 to 52,000 a year) – a far cry from the 20 cigs of an average tobacco smoker.

Smoked marijuana threatens patients with bacterial and fungal infections; it has been demonstrated that infectious agents can be found on marijuana leaves, [6] because it is clandestinely produced, and not subject to the obsessive quality controls that the targeted tobacco industry is. Cancer and AIDS patients are immuno-compromised and are extraordinarily sensitive to invasion by bacteria and fungi. [7] It is true that legalization would go toward eliminating this problem, but Mr. Sweanor certainly does not refer to any future.

According to a leading medical journal, marijuana users had 55% more industrial accidents than non-users. The same study found that marijuana users had 85% more injuries at work than non-users. [8] But there is positively no need for studies or medical skills to observe that marijuana decreases motor skills, concentration and coordination, and that accidents result from a distortion of time and space relationships. Not surprisingly, none of this is a problem for tobacco smokers, who do not fall into an idiotic, dumb stupor every time they light up. Furthermore, marijuana users have been shown to have a 78% increase in absenteeism over non-users. [9] If we want to legalize cannabis, let's do it for the right reasons of personal liberty and choice, and common sense -- not by hypocritically misrepresenting a narcotic as "good" (or at least "acceptable-because-it-is-better-than-tobacco"), not by exchanging one demon weed for another in a propaganda and junk science shell game.

How can we say that marijuana is not killing people? How much do we really know about it? Cannabis has been illegal for the last 70-100 years, depending on the country. If, for the sake of argument, marijuana kills slowly by creating disease conditions over decades, how could we possibly know about it? Cannabis is a major – although illicit -- cash crop for the Canadian province of British Columbia. How many people buying this product go around telling the neighbors, or confessing their consumption habits on the federal census? How many tell their own doctors?

The state cannot make money on this illegal substance through tax. Thus, marijuana – differently than tobacco -- has not attracted opportunistic scientists, Big Pharma, and so on to produce the mountain of junk science "evidence" about mortality and disease "attributions" on an industrial scale to get state grants, justify replacement "therapies," taxation increase, false propaganda, and all the rest of the mumbo jumbo that makes tobacco so lucrative today for the legions of hypocrites seeking to "control" it. There is no "marijuana industry" to sue, and to prey on with multibillion-dollar settlements. Tobacco smokers, however, who use a legal substance, can be easy targets of the social leaches of the antitobacco industry which, together with "public health," come one inch short of telling tobacco smokers to become marijuana smokers instead – presumably in order to be more socially acceptable. Once again, people who respect the law are the easy prey of the do-gooders.

Shame on you, Mr. Sweanor. Since you brought up the subject of defecation, we suggest that it is something that you stop doing to the truth. The personal and social consciences of a lot of antismokers seem to be comfortably numb - perhaps stoned permanently by what "is not killing people."

Gian Turci
FORCES International/Italy

[1] Yamamoto, et al. Pharm. Biochem. Behav. 40:465-469. 1991.

[2] Final Order of Administrator of DEA (Drug Enforcement Agency) denying the petition of NORML (National Organization for the Reform of Marijuana Laws) to reschedule the plant material marijuana from Schedule I to Schedule II of the Controlled Substances Act. Federal Register, V.54 #249, Dec. 29, 1989.

[3] Leveque, et al. HempTV transmission: "Marijuana and Medicine: Assessing the Science Base." The National Academy of Sciences, Institute of Medicine. Apr. 26, 1999.

[4] Starr, et al. Medical Tribune. Pg. 17. 1994.

[5] American Academy of Opthamology. The Use of Marijuana in the Treatment of Glaucoma. As cited at http://eyenet.org/public/glaucoma/gl_maryj.html. 1999.

APPENDIX F

Just to be Fair

Below is a web site with a list of references on articles opposing smoking. The site was working at the time of publication. It's enough to frighten anyone into quitting – even Humphrey Bogart and James Dean. You will note some legitimate medical journals among the references but the preponderance of the articles are from government sources (always suspect), public health departments (99.9 percent opposed to smoking in every shape or form, even if it is good for you in moderate amounts – We have an agenda; our careers depend on supporting it; we don't CARE about the science – unless it agrees with us.) and "private" societies such as the American Cancer Society, American Lung Association, the SPCA -- and Brooke Shields.

Not all of the 182 references are listed here, however you can find the web site and the complete list at http://www.quit.org.au/quit/FandI/welcome.htm then go to the "Table of Contents", then to "References to Chapter 3". Or enter the following web site: http://www.quit.org.au/quit/FandI/fandi/cr03.htm

Below are some excerpts from these references. You will note, there is NOT ONE that tells the other story and most of these simply **aren't true**, as the REAL scientific evidence suggests! They also don't give a hint as to the <u>healthful benefits of moderate inhalation of tobacco smoke</u>. So now you can read my book and the anti-tobacco references below, and make up your own mind.

- Nicotine, carbon monoxide and other toxic constituents of tobacco smoke cross the placenta readily, having a direct effect on the oxygen supply to the fetus, and the structure and function of the umbilical cord and placenta. A number of tobacco smoke constituents that cross the placenta are known carcinogens.

- Nicotine has a direct effect on fetal heart rate and breathing movements.

- Nicotine is also found in the breast milk of women who smoke.

- Spontaneous abortions and complications of pregnancy and labor occur more frequently in smokers.

- Smokers have a higher risk of ectopic (tubal) pregnancy and have a greater tendency to deliver preterm.

- Women who smoke during pregnancy have a 25 to 50% higher rate of fetal and infant deaths compared with non-smokers.

- Exposure by the mother to workplace passive smoking and paternal smoking has also been associated with lower birth weight, a higher risk of perinatal mortality and spontaneous abortion, particularly in the second trimester (mid three months) of pregnancy.

- Maternal smoking exerts a direct growth retarding effect on the fetus, resulting in a decrease in all dimensions including length and circumference of chest and head.

- Infants of smokers weigh on average 200 grams less than the infants of non-smokers, and smokers have double the risk of having a low birth weight baby.

- The mother smoked 5 or more cigarettes a day throughout the pregnancy. The mother had no evidence of hypertension during pregnancy, specifically no preeclampsia and documentation of normal blood pressure at least once after the first trimester.

- The newborn has symmetrical growth retardation at term, 37 weeks, defined as birth weight less than 2,500 grams, and a ponderal index (weight in grams divided by length) greater than 2.32. (Note: ponderal index is a measure used in Australia).

- There is no obvious cause of intrauterine growth retardation, that is, congenital malformation or infection."

- Maternal smoking may predispose the child to respiratory illness. Parental smoking has been linked with decreased pulmonary function and asthma in children.

- Smoking during pregnancy and in the infant's first year of life is considered one of the major risk factors for sudden infant death syndrome ('SIDS' or 'cot death')

- Research has suggested that smoking by either parent during pregnancy is associated with a higher incidence of all childhood cancers combined, but especially acute lymphocytic leukemia and lymphoma. There may be an association between paternal smoking and brain cancer.

- However at this stage, these findings are not consistent and should be considered as tentative.

- A recent meta-analysis suggests a small but statistically significant association between maternal cigarette smoking during the first trimester of pregnancy and increased risk of having a child with cleft lip/palate or cleft palate.

- Other reported long term effects of maternal smoking on the infant include impairment of behavioral, intellectual, and physical characteristics.

- A recent study found a strong and significant positive association between cigarette smoking in mothers during pregnancy and attention deficit/hyperactivity disorder in their children.

- See also Chapter 4 for discussion of the health effects of passive smoking for infants and children. Readers requiring more information are referred in the first instance to references and both of which provide fully referenced, recent reviews of the medical evidence on the effects of passive smoking on pregnancy and infancy.

List of Web Sites

Diseases

Impact of Smoking on Clinical and Angiographic Restenosis After Percutaneous Coronary Intervention http://193.78.190.200/34/circulation_2001_104_773.htm

This study shows yet another benefit of smoking. This time the benefit concerns restenosis, that is, the occlusion of coronary arteries. Smokers have much better chances to survive, heal and do well. Where is the press? Nowhere to be found, of course; we are talking about a significant positive effect of tobacco and smoking, which affects the health of people. Well, come on! We are also talking about *responsible media*, here... people increase their chances of death from cardiovascular disease by not smoking. Smoking, within certain limits, is good for your health– a totally unacceptable paradox.

Carbon Monoxide May Alleviate Heart Attacks And Stroke http://193.78.190.200/10b/cm.htm

Carbon monoxide is a by-product of tobacco smoke. A report indicates very low levels of carbon monoxide may help victims of heart attacks and strokes. Carbon monoxide inhibits blood clotting, thereby dissolving harmful clots in the arteries. The researchers focused on carbon monoxide's close resemblance to nitric oxide which keeps blood vessels from dilating and prevents the buildup of white blood cells. *"Recently nitric oxide has been elevated from a common air pollutant . . . to an [internal] second messenger of utmost physiological importance. Therefore, many of us may not be entirely surprised to learn that carbon monoxide can paradoxically rescue the lung from [cardiovascular blockage] injury."* The pharmacological benefits of tobacco are nothing new.

Research indicating that nicotine holds potential for non-surgical heart by-pass procedures honored by the American College of Cardiology
http://193.78.190.200/10/toben.htm

Dr. Christopher Heeschen of Stanford University was honored by the American College of Cardiology for his research on the effect of nicotine on angiogenesis (new blood vessel growth). His work took third place in the 2,000 entry Young Investigators Competition in the category of Physiology, Pharmacology and Pathology. Dr. Heeschen presented compelling data from research done at Stanford revealing that the simple plant protein, nicotine, applied in small harmless doses, produced new blood vessel growth around blocked arteries to oxygen-starved tissue.

Severe Gum Recession, Less Of A Risk For Smokers
http://193.78.190.200/10o/gums.htm

In the strange world that anti-tobacco has wrought, any research that deviates from the tobacco-is-the-root-of-all-evil template is noteworthy. Here is a study that shows that smokers are actually at lower risk from gum disease. This is one of the "Health Warnings" on cigarette packs in Canada. There is no solid proof for any of the diseases attributed to tobacco - just statistics and speculative associations, but the ministries of health continue to lie to the public, in a dazzling display of intellectual, professional, moral and political corruption.

Smoking Prevents Rare Skin Cancer
http://193.78.190.200/10b/kaposi.htm

A researcher at the National Cancer Institute is treading treacherous waters by suggesting that smoking may act as a preventive for developing a skin cancer that primarily afflicts elderly men in Mediterranean regions of Southern Italy, Greece and Israel (Kaposi's Sarcoma). Not that smoking should be recommended for that population, Dr. James Goedert is quick to assure his peers. What is important is not that smoking tobacco may help to prevent a rare form of cancer but that there is an admission by a researcher at the National Cancer Institute that there are ANY benefits to smoking.

Nitric oxide mediates a therapeutic effect of nicotine in ulcerative colitis
http://193.78.190.200/22/ncbi.htm

"CONCLUSIONS: Nicotine reduces circular muscle activity, predominantly through the release of nitric oxide-this appears to be 'up-regulated' in active ulcerative colitis. These findings may explain some of the therapeutic benefit from nicotine (and smoking) in ulcerative colitis and may account for the colonic motor dysfunction in active disease."

Twin Study Supports Protective Effect of Smoking For Parkinson's Disease
http://193.78.190.200/10m/twin.htm

"Dr. Tanner's group continued to see significant differences when dose was calculated until 10 years or 20 years prior to diagnosis. They conclude that this finding refutes the suggestion that individuals who smoke more are less likely to have PD because those who develop symptoms quit smoking. The inverse association of smoking dose and PD can be attributed to environmental, and not genetic, causes with near certainty," the authors write.' There has been a total silence from the antismoking mass media on this pivotal, long-range study that shows yet another benefit of smoking. If the intention of "public health" is to inform the public about the consequences of smoking on health as it proclaims, why don't we see "warnings" such as:

"Smoking Protects against Parkinson's Disease," or "Smoking protects against Alzheimer's Disease," or

"Smoking protects against Ulcerative Colitis" and so on, alongside with the other speculations on "tobacco-related" disease? Isn't the function of public health to tell the citizens about ALL the effects on health of a substance? "Public health," today, is nothing more than a deceiving propaganda machine paid by pharmaceutical and public money to promote frauds, fears, and puritanical rhetoric dressed up in white coats.

Shocker: "Villain" nicotine slays TB
http://193.78.190.200/10c/nicotine.htm

"Nicotine might be a surprising alternative someday for treating stubborn forms of tuberculosis, a University of Central Florida researcher said Monday. The compound stopped the growth of tuberculosis in laboratory tests, even when used in small quantities, said Saleh Naser, an associate professor of microbiology and molecular biology at UCF. ... Most scientists agree that nicotine is the substance that causes people to become addicted to cigarettes and other tobacco products." "... But no one is suggesting that people with TB take up the potentially deadly habit of smoking." Of course not. It is much better to develop medication-resistant superbugs than to start smoking...It should be said that the "most scientists" in question are paid off by the pharmaceutical industry for their research; and that most of the aforementioned "scientists" promote the nicotine-based "cessation" products manufactured by their masters -- mysteriously without explaining why such an addictive substance becomes *"un-addictive"* when used *to quit smoking!*

Parkinson's Disease Is Associated With Non-smoking
http://www.forces.org/evidence/carol/carol36.htm

Bibliography of references from studies associating Parkinson's disease with non-smoking. Certain benefits of smoking are well-documented, but the anti smoking groups, backed by several medical journals (more interested in advertising revenue than in informing the population), are silent. By the way, what about the *cost of non-smokers to society due to their prevailing tendency to contract Parkinson's disease?*

Alzheimer's Disease Is Associated With Non-Smoking http://www.forces.org/evidence/carol/carol16.htm

"A statistically significant inverse relation between smoking and Alzheimer's disease was observed at all levels of analysis, with a trend towards decreasing risk with increasing consumption".

Smokers have reduced risks of Alzheimer's and Parkinson's disease http://www.forces.org/evidence/files/liars.htm

Of the 19 studies, 15 found a reduce risk in smokers, and none found an increased risk. And smoking is clearly associated with a reduced risk of Parkinson's disease, another disease in which nicotine receptors are reduced. The fact that acute administration of nicotine improves attention and information processing in AD patients adds further plausibility to the hypothesis.

Nicotine Drugs Hold Promise for Treating Neurological Disease Alzheimer's patients may benefit, scientists say. http://193.78.190.200/10/nicoplus.htm

The anti-tobacco fanatics are in a tough spot. Reliable scientific research has turned up the horrible news that tobacco smoke is good for your health. Alzheimer's, Parkinson's, Tourette's Syndrome, and Senile Brain Disease are among some diseases that can be cured or alleviated by tobacco.

Women, Children and Tobacco

The Puzzling Association between Smoking and Hypertension during Pregnancy
http://193.78.190.200/2/14/ajog2.htm

This large study has examined nearly 10,000 pregnant women. Conclusion: *"Smoking is associated with a reduced risk of hypertension during pregnancy. The protective effect appears to continue even after cessation of smoking. Further basic research on this issue is warranted. (Am J Obstet Gynecol 1999;181:1407-13.)"*

For more information on smoking and pregnancy: http://www.forces.org/evidence/evid/preg.htm

Smoking: Protection Against Neural Tube Defects?
http://www.forces.org/evidence/files/neural.htm

Does tobacco smoke prevent atopic disorders? A study of two generations of Swedish residents
http://193.78.190.200/30/asthma.htm

"In a multivariate analysis, children of mothers who smoked at least 15 cigarettes a day tended to have lower odds for suffering from allergic rhino-conjunctivitis, allergic asthma, atopic eczema and food allergy, compared to children of mothers who had never smoked. Children of fathers who had smoked at least 15 cigarettes a day had a similar tendency)." Children of smokers have LOWER asthma! You certainly won't see this one on the health news of BBC or ABC, as they are too busy trying to convince us that smokers "cause" asthma in their kids - - and in the kids of others. That is not true, as smoking does not "cause" asthma.

Does maternal smoking hinder mother-child transmission of Helicobacter pylori infection
http://www.ncbi.nlm.nih.gov/entrez/query.fcgi?db=

PubMed&cmd=Retrieve&list_uids=10615847&dopt=Abstract

"Evidence for early childhood as the critical period of Helicobacter pylori infection and for clustering of the infection within families suggests a major role of intrafamilial transmission. In a previous study, we found a strong inverse relation between maternal smoking and H. pylori infection among preschool children, suggesting the possibility that mother-child transmission of the infection may be less efficient if the mother smokes. To evaluate this hypothesis further, we carried out a subsequent population-based study in which H. pylori infection was measured by 13C-urea breath test in 947 preschool children and their mothers. We obtained detailed information on potential risk factors for infection, including maternal smoking, by standardized questionnaires. Overall, 9.8% (93 of 947) of the children and 34.7% (329 of 947) of the mothers were infected. Prevalence of infection was much lower among children of uninfected mothers (1.9%) than among children of infected mothers (24.7%). There was a strong inverse relation of children's infection with maternal smoking (adjusted odds ratio = 0.24; 95% confidence interval = 0.12-0.49) among children of infected mothers, but not among children of uninfected mothers. These results support the hypothesis of a predominant role for mother-child transmission of H. pylori infection, which may be less efficient if the mother smokes.".

For more information on smoking and pregnancy go to: http://www.forces.org/evidence/evid/preg.htm

Risk of papillary thyroid cancer in women in relation to smoking and alcohol consumption
http://www.aim-digest.com/gateway/pages/cancer/articles/papill.htm

"Both smoking and alcohol consumption may influence thyroid function, although the nature of these relations is not well understood. We examined the influence of tobacco and alcohol use on risk of papillary thyroid cancer in a population-based case-control study. Of 558 women with thyroid cancer diagnosed during 1988-1994 identified as eligible, 468 (83.9%) were interviewed; this analysis was restricted to women with papillary histology (N = 410). Controls (N = 574) were identified by random digit dialing, with a response proportion of 73.6%. We used logistic regression to calculate odds ratios (OR) and associated confidence intervals (CI) estimating the relative risk of papillary thyroid cancer associated with cigarette smoking and alcohol consumption. A history of ever having smoked more than 100 cigarettes was associated with a reduced risk of disease (OR = 0.7, 95% CI = 0.5-0.9). This reduction in risk was most evident in current smokers (OR = 0.5, 95% CI = 0.4-0.7). Women who reported that they had ever consumed 12 or more alcohol-containing drinks within a year were also at reduced risk (OR 0.7, 95% CI = 0.5-1.0). Similar to the association noted with smoking, the reduction in risk was primarily present among current alcohol consumers. The associations we observed, if not due to chance, may be related to actions of cigarette smoking and alcohol consumption that reduce thyroid cell proliferation through effects on thyroid stimulating hormone, estrogen, or other mechanisms."

Urinary Cotinine Concentration Confirms the Reduced Risk of Preeclampsia with Tobacco Exposure
http://193.78.190.200/2/13/ajog.htm

This study, though small, shows one of the benefits of smoking during pregnancy. *"These findings, obtained by using laboratory assay, confirm the reduced risk of developing preeclampsia with tobacco exposure. (Am J Obstet Gynecol 1999;181:1192-6.*

For more information on smoking and pregnancy go to: http://www.forces.org/evidence/evid/preg.htm

Smoking Reduces The Risk Of Breast Cancer
http://www.forces.org/evidence/files/brea.htm

A new study in the *Journal of the National Cancer Institute* (May 20, 1998) reports that carriers of a particular gene mutation (which predisposes the carrier to breast cancer) who smoked cigarettes for more than 4 pack years (i.e., number of packs per day multiplied by the number of years of smoking) were found to have a statistically significant 54 percent decrease in breast cancer incidence when compared with carriers who never smoked. One strength of the study is that the reduction in incidence exceeds the 50 percent threshold. However, we think it important to point out that this was a small, case control study (only 300 cases) based on self-reported data.

Effects of Transdermal Nicotine on Cognitive Performance in Down's Syndrome
http://193.78.190.200/13/tlj.htm

"We investigated the effect of nicotine-agonistic stimulation with 5 mg transdermal patches, compared with placebo, on cognitive performance in five adults with the disorder. Improvements possibly related to attention and information processing were seen for Down's syndrome patients compared with healthy controls. Our preliminary findings are encouraging..." More benefits of nicotine. Of course, it is politically incorrect to say that this is a benefit of *smoking* - only of the pharmaceutically-produced transdermal nicotine, the one that is terribly addictive if delivered through cigarettes, but not addictive at all, and even *beneficial*, when delivered through patches.... Antismoking nonsense aside, nicotine gets into the

body regardless of the means of delivery. And more evidence about the benefis seems to emerge quite often, though the small size of this study cannot certainly be taken as conclusive.

Miscellaneous

Nicotine Benefits   http://www.forces.org/evidence/hamilton/other/nicotine.htm

The benefits of nicotine -- and smoking -- are described in this bibliography. This information is an example of what the anti-tobacco groups do not want publicized because it fails to support their agenda. Some of the studies report benefits not just from nicotine, but from *smoking itself*. But of course, according to the anti-smokers, all these scientists have been "paid by the tobacco industry" ... even though this is not true. Sadly, personal slander and misinformation are the price a scientist has to pay for honest work on tobacco.

Smoking Your Way to Good Health
http://193.78.190.200/10/nicoplus.htm

The benefits of smoking tobacco have been common knowledge for centuries. From sharpening mental acuity to maintaining optimal weight, the relatively small risks of smoking have always been outweighed by the substantial improvement to mental and physical health. Hysterical attacks on tobacco notwithstanding, smokers always weigh the good against the bad and puff away or quit according to their personal preferences. Now the same anti-tobacco enterprise that has spent billions demonizing the pleasure of smoking is providing additional reasons to smoke. Alzheimer's, Parkinson's, Tourette's Syndrome, even schizophrenia and cocaine addiction are disorders that are alleviated by tobacco. Add in the still inconclusive indication that tobacco helps to prevent colon and prostate cancer and the endorsement for smoking tobacco by the medical establishment is good news for smokers and non-smokers alike. Of course the revelation that tobacco is good for you is ruined by the pharmaceutical industry's plan to substitute the natural and relatively inexpensive tobacco plant with their overpriced and ineffective nicotine substitutions. Still, when all is said and done, the positive revelations regarding tobacco are very good reasons indeed to keep lighting those cigarettes.

The Carbon Monoxide Paradox
http://193.78.190.200/10b/cm.htm

A killer gas may actually be a lifesaver, surprising research in mice, reveals.

Theraputic effects of Nicotine and Smoking http://www.forces.org/evidence/evid/therap.htm The following quote is a good summary of the illogical and dishonest media the smoker faces: "Since the benefits of smoking are too numerous and consistent to be attributable to error or random chance, it follows that the "established truth" asserting that smoking is the cause of (almost) all disease cannot be true - a reality that dramatically clashes with the gigantic corruption of public health, it's pharmaceutical and insurance mentors, institutions and media." (Quoted from *Forces*, the British defenders of the right to smoke).

Must Reading for Those Interested in Personal Liberty (whether you smoke or not)

For Your Own Good – Jacob Sullum, The free press, N.Y., 1998.

You will get a sense of the impending Nazi-like future we are facing from reading this book. Sullum doesn't exactly say that, but it's the message as I see it. I think the trend is unstoppable but you should read this book, so that someday you can explain to your grand-children how things went wrong.

Passive Smoke – Gori and Luik, Fraser Institute, Vancouver, B.C., 1999.

The greatest science swindle of all time by an official arm of the U.S. Government, the Environmental Protection agency, is clearly explained down to the level of the most fanatic pinko moron in the anti-smoking movement. It is an ugly tale of deceit, data manipulation, and venality that prove "government science" to be the perfect example of an oxymoron.

Slow Burn – Don Oakley, Eyrie Press, Roswell, GA. This book is more in line with my approach but with a little more on statistics. Don't let that frighten you away. This book is humorous, deadly logical, and full of interesting quotes and important data. It is better than my book and I cribbed a lot of useful information out of it.

About
William Campbell Douglass, II MD

Consumed by a passion for living a long healthy life, Dr. Douglass has spent over 40 years swimming against the current of popular medical propaganda. He is unwavering in his dedication to improving the quality of life of his readers. Dr. Douglass has been called "the conscience of modern medicine," a "medical maverick," and has been voted "Doctor of the Year" by the National Health Federation.

His medical experiences read like an Indiana Jones novel, from battling malaria in Central America, fighting deadly epidemics at his own health clinic in Africa, flying with U.S. Navy crews as a flight surgeon, and saving lives for over a decade in emergency medicine. This dedicated physician has repeatedly gone far beyond the call of duty in his work to spread the truth about alternative therapies.

For a full year, he endured economic and physical hardship while working on photoluminescence research with physicians at the Pasteur Institute in St. Petersburg Russia. These learning experiences, not to mention his keen storytelling ability and wit, make Dr. Douglass' newsletters and all of his books uniquely interesting and fun to read.

Dr. William C. Douglass has led a colorful, rebellious, and crusading life. Not many physicians would dare put their professional reputations on the line as many times as this courageous healer has. A vocal opponent of "business-as-usual" medicine, Dr. Douglass has championed patients' rights and physician commitment to wellness throughout his career. He comes from a distinguished family of physicians. Dr. Douglass graduated from the University of Rochester, the Miami School of Medicine, the Naval School of Aviation and Space Medicine and is the fourth generation Douglass to practice medicine.

Dr. Douglass has two adult children. His son, "Camp", lives in Florida and is also a doctor and his daughter, Tracy, is a television personality and researcher and editor for her father. Dr. Douglass lives abroad with his wife Melissa and their Weimaraner dog "Silky".

Index

C

D

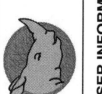

Rhino Publishing, S.A.

Fax a copy of this order to:
1-888-317-6767 or Int'l + 416-352-5126

ORDER FORM

Rhino Publishing, S.A. Attention: PTY 5048
P.O. Box 025724, Miami, FL. 33102 USA

PURCHASER INFORMATION

Purchaser's Name (Please Print): _____

Shipping Address (Do not use a P.O. Box): _____

City: _____ State/Prov.: _____ Country: _____

Zip/Postal Code: _____ Telephone No.: _____ Fax No.:: _____

Special Instructions for delivery: _____

E-Mail Address (if interested in receiving free e-Books when available): _____

CREDIT CARD INFO: AMERICAN EXPRESS, DISCOVER, MASTERCARD AND VISA ONLY

Name on the Card: _____ Type of Card: _____

Charge my Card ⮞ Number #: _____ Exp.: _____

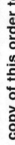

*Security Code: _____ * Required for all MasterCard, Visa and American Express purchases. For your security, we require that you enter your card's verification number. The verification number is also called a CCV number. This code is the 3 digits farthest right in the signature field on the back of your VISA/MC, or the 4 digits to the right on the front of your American Express card. Your credit card statement will show a **different name than Rhino Publishing** as the vendor.

If your shipping address is not the same as your credit card billing address, please indicate your card billing address here.

Billing Address: _____

City: _____ State/Prov.: _____ Zip/Postal Code: _____

Country: _____

Fax a copy of this order with your credit card information to:
1-888-317-6767 or International #: + 416-352-5126

To order by mail, send your payment by first class mail only to the following address.
Include a copy of this order form.

Please make your check or bank drafts (NO postal money order please)
payable to RHINO PUBLISHING, S.A. and mail to:

Attention: PTY 5048
P.O. Box 025724
Miami, FL.
USA 33102

Digital E-books also available online: www.rhinopublish.com

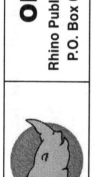

Rhino Publishing, S.A.

Fax a copy of this order to:
1-888-317-6767 or Int'l + 416-352-5126

ORDER FORM

Rhino Publishing, S.A. Attention: PTY 5048
P.O. Box 025724, Miami, FL. 33102 USA

Purchaser's Name (Please Print): _____ Tel.: _____

Health Books

			Rhino Special Price
___	X	9962-636-04-3	Add 10 Years to Your Life (Retail: $15.99)	X $13.99 = $ ___
___	X	9962-636-07-8	AIDS and Biological Warfare (Retail: $22.99)	X $17.99 = $ ___
___	X	9962-636-09-4	Bad Medicine (Retail: $13.99)	X $11.99 = $ ___
___	X	9962-636-10-8	Color Me Healthy (Retail: $13.99)	X $11.99 = $ ___
___	X	9962-636-XX-X	Color Me Healthy 11 Roscolene Filters 4" X 4" (Retail: $21.89)	X $20.00 = $ ___
___	X	9962-636-YY-Y	Color Me Healthy 11 Roscolene Filters 6.5" X 6.5" (Retail: $36.89)	X $30.00 = $ ___
___	X	9962-636-ZZ-Z	Color Me Healthy 11 Roscolene Filters 8" X 8" (Retail: $51.89)	X $40.00 = $ ___
___	X	9962-636-15-9	Dangerous Legal Drugs (Retail: $15.99)	X $13.99 = $ ___
___	X	9962-636-18-3	Dr. Douglass' Complete Guide to Better Vision (Retail: $13.99)	X $11.99 = $ ___
___	X	9962-636-19-1	Eat Your Cholesterol! (Retail: $13.99)	X $11.99 = $ ___
___	X	9962-636-12-4	Grandma Bell's A To Z Guide To Healing (Retail: $17.99)	X $14.99 = $ ___
___	X	9962-636-22-1	Hormone Replacement Therapies (Retail: $13.99)	X $11.99 = $ ___
___	X	9962-636-25-6	Hydrogen Peroxide. Medical Miracle (Retail: $18.99)	X $15.99 = $ ___
___	X	9962-636-27-2	Into the Light (Retail: $25.99)	X $19.99 = $ ___

X 9962-636-32-9 Prostate Problems (Retail: $13.99)   X $13.99 = $

___ X 9962-636-34-5 St. Petersburg Nights (Retail: $22.99)   X $17.99 = $
___ X 9962-636-37-X Stop Aging or Slow the Process (Retail: $13.99)   X $11.99 = $
___ X 9962-636-60-4 The Hypertension Report (Retail: $13.99)   X $11.99 = $
___ X 9962-636-48-5 The Joy of Mature Sex (Retail: $15.99)   X $13.99 = $
___ X 9962-636-43-4 The Health Benefits of Tobacco (Retail: $29.99)   X $22.99 = $

Political Books:

___ X 9962-636-40-X The Eagle's Feather (Retail: $19.99)   X $15.99 = $
___ X 9962-636-40-X The Hemp Conspiracy by Paul Wylie (Retail: $22.99)   X $17.99 = $
___ X 9962-636-00-0 Painful Dilemma, Patients in Pain - People in Prison (Retail: $22.99)   X $17.99 = $
___ X 9962-636-32-9 Prostate Problems (Retail: $13.99)   X $11.99 = $

                                                                    SUB-TOTAL............. $

ADD $5.00 HANDLING FOR YOUR ORDER: $5.00 = $ 5.00

ADD $2.50 SHIPPING FOR EACH ITEM ON ORDER: + ___ X $2.50 = $

NOTE THAT THE MINIMUM SHIPPING AND HANDLING IS $7.50 FOR 1 BOOK ($5.00 + $2.50)
Or for order shipped outside the US, add $5.00 per item

ADD $5.00 S. & H. OR EACH ITEM ON ORDER (INTERNATIONAL ORDERS ONLY)   + ___ X $5.00 = $

Allow up to 21 days for delivery (we will call you about back orders if any)

                                                           TOTAL PAID............. $

Digital E-books also available online: www.rhinopublish.com

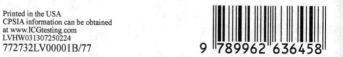

9 789962 636458